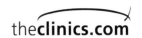
theclinics.com

ANESTHESIOLOGY CLINICS

Influence of Perioperative
Care on Outcome

GUEST EDITOR
Steffen E. Meiler, MD

CONSULTING EDITOR
Lee A. Fleisher, MD

June 2006 • Volume 24 • Number 2

SAUNDERS

An Imprint of Elsevier, Inc.
PHILADELPHIA   LONDON   TORONTO   MONTREAL   SYDNEY   TOKYO

W.B. SAUNDERS COMPANY
A Division of Elsevier Inc.

1600 John F. Kennedy Boulevard, Suite 1800 • Philadelphia, Pennsylvania 19103-2899

http://www.theclinics.com

ANESTHESIOLOGY CLINICS
June 2006
Editor: Rachel Glover

Volume 24, Number 2
ISSN 0889-8537
ISBN 1-4160-3572-9

The ideas and opinions expressed in *Anesthesiology Clinics* do not necessarily reflect those of the Publisher. The Publisher does not assume any responsibility for any injury and/or damage to persons or property arising out of or related to any use of the material contained in this periodical. The reader is advised to check the appropriate medical literature and the product information currently provided by the manufacturer of each drug to be administered to verify the dosage, the method and duration of administration, or contraindications. It is the responsibility of the treating physician or other health care professional, relying on independent experience and knowledge of the patient, to determine drug dosages and the best treatment for the patient. Mention of any product in this issue should not be construed as endorsement by the contributors, editors, or the Publisher of the product or manufacturers' claims.

Anesthesiology Clinics (ISSN 0889-8537) is published quarterly by W.B. Saunders, 360 Park Avenue South, New York, NY 10010-1710. Months of publication are March, June, September, December. Business and Editorial Offices: 1600 John F. Kennedy Blvd., Suite 1800, Philadelphia, PA 19103-2899. Accounting and Circulation Offices: 6277 Sea Harbor Drive, Orlando, FL 32887-4800. Periodicals postage paid at New York, NY and additional mailing offices. Subscription prices are $90.00 per year (US student/resident), $180.00 per year (US individuals), $220.00 per year (Canadian individuals), $285.00 per year (US institutions), $345.00 per year (Canadian institutions), $235.00 per year (foreign individuals), and $345.00 per year (foreign institutions). To receive student and resident rate, orders must be accompanied by name of affiliated institution, date of term, and the *signature* of program/residency coordinator on institutions letterhead. Orders will be billed at individual rate until proof of status is received. Foreign air speed delivery is included in all *Clinics'* subscription prices. All prices are subject to change without notice. POSTMASTER: Send address changes to *Anesthesiology Clinics*, Elsevier Periodicals Customer Service, 6277 Sea Harbor Drive, Orlando, FL 32887-4800. Customer Service: 1-800-654-2452 (US). From outside of the US, call 1-407-345-4000. E-mail: hhspcs@wbsaunders.com.

Anesthesiology Clinics is also published in Spanish by McGraw-Hill Inter-americana Editores S. A., P.O. Box 5-237, 06500 Mexico D. F., Mexico.

Anesthesiology Clinics is covered in *Index Medicus, Current Contents/Clinical Medicine, Excerpta Medica, ISI/BIOMED*, and *Chemical Abstracts*.

Printed in the United States of America.

CONSULTING EDITOR

LEE A. FLEISHER, MD, Robert D. Dripps Professor and Chair, Department of Anesthesiology and Critical Care and Medicine, University of Pennsylvania School of Medicine, Philadelphia, Pennsylvania

GUEST EDITOR

STEFFEN E. MEILER, MD, Associate Professor of Anesthesiology and Medicine; Vice Chair of Research; Director, Program of Molecular Perioperative Medicine & Genomics, Medical College of Georgia, Augusta, Georgia

CONTRIBUTORS

STIG BENGMARK, MD, PhD, FRACS (hon), FRCPS (hon); Fellow, Academia Europeae; Emeritus Professor, Lund University, Lund, Sweden; Honorary Visiting Professor, Departments of Hepatology and Surgery, University College London, London, United Kingdom

ANGELIKA BIERHAUS, Department of Medicine I, University of Heidelberg, Heidelberg, Germany

ANNA CARNINI, PhD, Postdoctoral Fellow, Department of Anesthesiology and Critical Care, University of Pennsylvania Health Systems, Philadelphia, Pennsylvania

MARCEL E. DURIEUX, MD, PhD, Professor of Anesthesiology and Neurological Surgery, University of Virginia Medical Center, Charlottesville, Virginia

MARYELLEN FAZEN ECKENHOFF, PhD, Research Associate, Department of Anesthesiology and Critical Care, University of Pennsylvania Health Systems, Philadelphia, Pennsylvania

RODERIC G. ECKENHOFF, MD, Lamont Professor and Vice Chair for Research, Department of Anesthesiology and Critical Care, University of Pennsylvania Health Systems, Philadelphia, Pennsylvania

PER M. HUMPERT, Department of Medicine I, University of Heidelberg, Heidelberg, Germany

SHUKRI F. KHURI, MD, Professor of Surgery, Harvard Medical School, Boston, Massachusetts; Chief, Cardiothoracic Surgery, VA Boston Healthcare System, West Roxbury, Massachusetts

JAMES B. MAYFIELD, MD, Assistant Professor and Vice Chair, Clinical Anesthesia, Department of Anesthesiology and Perioperative Medicine; Director, Perioperative Services, Medical College of Georgia, Augusta, Georgia

STEFFEN E. MEILER, MD, Associate Professor of Anesthesiology and Medicine; Vice Chair of Research; Director, Program of Molecular Perioperative Medicine & Genomics, Medical College of Georgia, Augusta, Georgia

PETER P. NAWROTH, Department of Medicine I, University of Heidelberg, Heidelberg, Germany

CHARLES N. SERHAN, PhD, Simon Gelman Professor of Anaesthesia (Biochemistry and Molecular Pharmacology), Brigham and Women's Hospital and Harvard Medical School; Professor and Head, Department of Oral Medicine, Infection and Immunity, Harvard School of Dental Medicine, Boston Massachusetts

DANIEL I. SESSLER, MD, Chair, Department of Outcomes Research, Cleveland Clinic Foundation; Cleveland, Ohio; L&S Weakley Professor of Anesthesiology and Director, Outcomes Research Institute, University of Louisville, Louisville, Kentucky

ASHLEY M. SHILLING, MD, Assistant Professor of Anesthesiology, University of Virginia Medical Center, Charlottesville, Virginia

ROBERT K. STOELTING, MD, President, Anesthesia Patient Safety Foundation, Indianapolis, Indiana

CONTENTS

> Anesthesiology has served as a model for patient safety in health care
> and was the first medical profession to treat patient safety as an inde-
> pendent problem. Anesthesiology has implemented widely accepted
> guidelines on basic monitoring, conducted long-term analyses of
> closed malpractice claims, developed patient simulators as meaning-
> ful training tools, and addressed problems of human error. The
> National Surgical Quality Improvement Program is the first national,
> validated, and peer-controlled program that uses risk-adjusted
> outcomes for the comparative assessment and improvement of the
> quality of surgical care. The program has reduced postoperative com-
> plications in the Veterans Administration, at both national and local
> levels. It is becoming more evident that processes and events during
> surgery can be important determinants of long-term outcomes after
> anesthesia and surgery.

> There is a strong possibility that the risk from anesthesia and sur-
> gery carries over from the immediate perioperative period to more
> remote time points. This extended risk seems to influence the pro-
> gression, severity, and complication rate of certain chronic illnesses.
> With the recognition that the perioperative process could be
> responsible for later adverse events comes the need to reassess

existing patient safety models, because some of the risk could be preventable. In the meantime, we must strive to improve short- and long-term outcomes by expanding our efforts to reduce disease activity preoperatively, to control the surgical stress response and infection rate, and to use tissue-preserving surgical techniques.

Non-pharmacologic Prevention of Surgical Wound Infection 279
Daniel I. Sessler

Wound infections are relatively common postoperative complications that are generally detected 5 to 9 days after surgery. Adequacy of host immune defenses is the primary factor that determines whether wound contamination progresses into a clinical infection. Many determinants of infection risk are under the direct control of anesthesiologists; factors that are at least as important as prophylactic antibiotics. This article reviews non-pharmacologic methods of reducing infection risk, including studies that demonstrate the benefits of keeping patients normothermic and supplying supplemental oxygen during surgery.

Bioecologic Control of Inflammation and Infection in Critical Illness 299
Stig Bengmark

Surgical and medical emergencies and treatments are still affected by an unacceptably high rate of morbidity and mortality. Sepsis is the most common medical and surgical complication and the tenth most common cause of death. Antibiotics and antagonists and inhibitors of proinflammatory cytokines have not met expectations. Selective bowel decontamination is no longer a treatment option. After more than 30 randomized clinical trials and 30 years of dedicated efforts to combat sepsis by the use of various combinations of antibiotics, we seem ready to conclude that the vigorous use of antibiotics does not significantly reduce mortality in critically ill patients. Side effects and price constitute important obstacles, especially when it comes to use of cytokine antagonists and inhibitors.

Linking Stress to Inflammation 325
Angelika Bierhaus, Per M. Humpert, and Peter P. Nawroth

Acute and chronic psychosocial stress leads to the activation of leukocytes and inflammatory reflexes, resulting in metabolic changes. These cellular responses contribute to the finding, that psychosocial stress is an independent predictor of mortality. This article links the current knowledge on inflammatory reactions induced by psychosocial stress to metabolic and vascular disease.

some disease-causing proteins, notably the amyloid β peptide of Alzheimer's disease. Although data in support of an interaction in the many available animal models are still lacking, data from clinical studies support an association, which provides further cause for concern. Many opportunities exist for rapid progress at all levels on defining whether anesthetics do indeed contribute to the pathogenesis of these progressive, debilitating disorders.

A common goal among physicians and nurses who practice anesthesia is to make surgery and anesthesia as safe as possible. In the modern practice of anesthesiology, many different monitors are used to acquire essential information to enhance patient care. We routinely rely on sophisticated monitors to ensure adequate function of anesthesia machines and assess physiologic function and depth of anesthesia. The question as to whether any of our intraoperative monitors have impact on patient safety has gained considerable attention in recent years. Physicians monitor patients to recognize and evaluate potential physiologic problems and identify prognostic trends. Although it is rational to believe that improved monitoring should reduce risk and increase patient safety, we must look critically at the evidence.

FORTHCOMING ISSUES

September 2006
Common Medical Conditions and Anesthesia
Stanley H. Rosenbaum, MD, *Guest Editor*

December 2006
Monitoring
Jeffrey S. Vender, MD, *Guest Editor*

RECENT ISSUES

March 2006
Palliative Care
Jonathan R. Gavrin, MD, *Guest Editor*

December 2005
Pediatric Anesthesiology
Andrew T. Costarino Jr, MD, and
B. Randall Brenn, MD, *Guest Editors*

September 2005
Obesity and Sleep Apnea
Peter Rock, MD, MBA, FCCP, FCCM, *Guest Editor*

THE CLINICS ARE NOW AVAILABLE ONLINE!

For more information about Clinics:
http://www.theclinics.com

ELSEVIER
SAUNDERS

Anesthesiology Clin N Am
24 (2006) xi–xii

ANESTHESIOLOGY
CLINICS OF
NORTH AMERICA

Foreword

Influence of Perioperative Care on Outcome

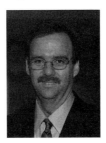

Lee A. Fleisher, MD
Consulting Editor

Over the past several years, there has been a small but growing series of papers that suggest that management decisions made during the perioperative period may influence outcomes long after surgery. These provocative papers led to the convening of a meeting by the Anesthesia Patient Safety Foundation. At that meeting, both the data and potential mechanisms were discussed. Although highly provocative, additional research is clearly required to determine if the link truly exists, and if so, how best to modify that risk. Those of us who attended the meeting believed that the information presented would be useful to all anesthesiologists, leading to the development of this issue of the *Anesthesiology Clinics of North America*.

Steffen E. Meiler, MD was a clear choice for editor of this issue. His major area of interest is the perioperative immune response. He is currently Vice Chairman of Research and Director of the Program for Molecular Perioperative Medicine & Genomics at the Medical College of Georgia. As one of those who attended the original meeting, he was able to assemble this international group of investigators to produce an outstanding issue that should stimulate those interested in this area for many years to come.

0889-8537/06/$ – see front matter © 2006 Elsevier Inc. All rights reserved.
doi:10.1016/j.atc.2006.03.004   *anesthesiology.theclinics.com*

Lee A. Fleisher, MD
Department of Anesthesiology and Critical Care
University of Pennsylvania School of Medicine
3400 Spruce Street
Philadelphia, PA 19104, USA
E-mail address: Lee.fleisher@uphs.upenn.edu

ELSEVIER
SAUNDERS

Anesthesiology Clin N Am
24 (2006) xiii–xiv

ANESTHESIOLOGY
CLINICS OF
NORTH AMERICA

Preface

Influence of Perioperative Care on Outcome

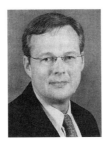

Steffen E. Meiler, MD
Guest Editor

After surgery, it was once thought, those patients who fared better simply tended to be those free of preexisting conditions. However, accumulating evidence shows that care decisions and events around the time of surgery not only influence patient outcome, but that they do so far after the perioperative period. These insights have informed recent patient safety initiatives and have attracted the attention of both health care providers and research scientists. They are of particular interest to anesthesiologists, inasmuch as they both redefine the impact that we as anesthesiologists can have on our patients in the short time that we care for them, and require us to explore in much more depth the effects of the perioperative process on surgical outcome. If we are successfully to meet this challenge by developing novel therapies and further improving the health care process, we must engage in constructive dialogs across our respective specialties.

This collection of monographs was designed to do exactly that—to convene national experts from patient safety organizations in anesthesia and surgery, clinical experts, and renowned scientists from diverse backgrounds to survey the larger organizational challenges, recent clinical progress, and the biology of this important area. Stressing the need for a joint approach, the opening article of this issue communicates the accomplishments, recent progress, and the future of patient safety from the perspective of the Anesthesia Patient Safety Foundation and the National Surgical Quality Improvement Program. To reflect the growing awareness of the role of the immune system in determining patient outcome,

doi:10.1016/j.atc.2006.03.003
anesthesiology.theclinics.com

special emphasis has been placed on inflammation, inflammation resolution, and immunity in the context of stress, nutrition, infection control, and other perioperative variables. Equally pertinent, however, are the discussions of pharmacological strategies for cardiac risk reduction, the potential association between volatile anesthetics and neurodegenerative diseases, and the impact of intraoperative monitoring on patient safety. It is our hope that this issue of the *Anesthesiology Clinics of North America* will begin to map this exciting new frontier, encouraging further explorations by research scientists and clinicians alike.

Steffen E. Meiler, MD
Medical College of Georgia
Department of Anesthesiology and Perioperative Medicine
1120 15th Street, BIW 2144
Augusta, GA 30912, USA
E-mail address: smeiler@mcg.edu

ELSEVIER
SAUNDERS

Anesthesiology Clin N Am
24 (2006) 235–253

ANESTHESIOLOGY
CLINICS OF
NORTH AMERICA

Past Accomplishments and Future Directions: Risk Prevention in Anesthesia and Surgery

Robert K. Stoelting, MD[a],*, Shukri F. Khuri, MD[b]

[a]*Anesthesia Patient Safety Foundation, 8007 South Meridian Street, Building One, Suite 2, Indianapolis, IN 46217, USA*
[b]*VA Boston Healthcare System, 1400 V.F.W. Parkway, West Roxbury, MA 02132, USA*

Anesthesiology was the first medical specialty to recognize patient safety as an independent problem [1]. The coincidence of multiple factors in the late 1970s led to significant changes in anesthesia practice that contributed to the decrease in mortality and catastrophic morbidity associated with adverse anesthesia-related events [2,3]. Although the magnitude of this decrease in anesthesia mortality is difficult to verify and anesthesia-related mortality still occurs, it is clear that anesthesia for healthy patients is safer today than it was in the past [4–6].

Anesthesia patient safety movement

In 1984, Ellison C. Pierce, Jr., MD, was president of the American Society of Anesthesiologists (ASA), and he formed the ASA Committee on Patient Safety and Risk Management, which emphasized the need to address the causes of patient injury related to administration of anesthesia. Around this same time, national media described anesthesia injuries that resulted in mobilization of public opinion for action [7], and professional liability insurance premiums for anesthesiologists escalated. Thus, the stage was set for creation of the Anesthesia Patient Safety Foundation (APSF) in 1985 under the direction of Dr. Pierce and with the administrative and financial support of the ASA [8,9].

* Corresponding author.
E-mail address: rstoelting@aol.com (R.K. Stoelting).

0889-8537/06/$ – see front matter. Published by Elsevier Inc.
doi:10.1016/j.atc.2006.01.004

Anesthesia Patient Safety Foundation

APSF functions as an independent nonprofit foundation which is guided by the mission "that no patient shall be harmed by anesthesia [8,9]." APSF is unique in that it brings together all stakeholders in patient safety including anesthesiologists, certified registered nurse anesthetists, pharmaceutical and device risk managers, attorneys, insurers, and representatives from the Food and Drug Administration (FDA), Joint Commission on Accreditation of Health Care Organizations (JCAHO), the American College of Surgeons (ACS), and the American Medical Association (AMA). The neutral umbrella of APSF facilitates open communication about the sensitive issues of anesthesia accidents. APSF has sponsored patient safety research, and the *APSF Newsletter* of current safety information reaches 75,000 worldwide, including every member of the ASA and American Association of Nurse Anesthetists (AANA), as well as corporate sponsors.

Public recognition

The success of the anesthesia patient safety movement was recognized in 1996 when the American Medical Association and corporate partners founded the National Patient Safety Foundation, which was based on the APSF model. Further recognition for safety efforts and leadership came to APSF in the landmark 1999 report from the Institute of Medicine (IOM) on errors in medical care [2]. In 2005, *The Wall Street Journal* carried a front page article about the successful efforts of anesthesiologists, the ASA, and APSF to improve anesthesia patient safety.

Culture of safety

In the long-term, the most important contribution of anesthesiology to patient safety may be the institutionalization and legitimization of patient safety as a topic of professional concern [1]. In this regard, the creation of APSF was a landmark achievement. Unlike professional societies such as ASA, APSF can bring together many constituencies in health care that may well disagree over economic (industry competitors) or political issues, but which all agree on the goal of patient safety.

Anesthesia is now safer

It is widely believed that anesthesia is safer today (at least for healthy patients) than it was 25 to 50 years ago, although the extent of and reasons for the improvements are debatable [4–6]. Traditional epidemiological studies on the incidence of adverse anesthesia events often cannot be compared because of different analysis techniques and inconsistent definitions of adverse events. An important result of this problem is the emergence of investigative techniques that do not focus on the incidence of an event but rather the underlying characteristics of mishaps (root cause analysis) and the attempt to improve subsequent patient care so that similar accidents do not recur. Examples of this approach include critical incident analysis and the analysis of closed malpractice claims by the ASA [1,10]. These approaches analyze only a small proportion of events that occur but attempt to extract the maximum amount of valuable information.

Improved patient safety

Technological improvements

In the early 1980s, important advances in technology became available. Electronic monitoring (inspired oxygen concentrations, pulse oximetry, capnography) that extended the human senses facilitated reliable, real-time, and continuous monitoring of oxygen delivery and patient oxygenation and ventilation. Although these monitors are believed to improve patient safety, no study has proved an outcome benefit from the use of these technologies. However, evidence from randomized controlled studies may neither be necessary nor appropriate for all interventions needed to improve patient safety [3]. With respect to modern knowledge about how complex systems get safer, the relentless and uncritical requirement of formal scientific proof lacks validity [3].

Another technological strategy is the use of engineered safety devices that physically prevent errors from occurring [1]. An example of this human factor design is the system of gas connectors that prevent a gas hose or cylinder from being connected to the incorrect site. New technologies have been developed to managing the patient's airway, including laryngeal mask airways and the fiberoptic laryngoscope, which results in improved management of the airway in both routine and emergency conditions. The FDA's anesthesia apparatus checkout recommendations were widely adopted. Improvements in the pharmacokinetics of anesthesia drugs have resulted in more specific and controllable pharmacological actions and fewer dangerous side effects.

Standards and guidelines

In the early 1980s a committee at the Harvard Hospitals proposed the first standards of practice for minimum intra-operative monitoring that became the forerunner of the ASA Standards on Basic Anesthetic Monitoring which were adopted in 1986. Continued revisions include the recent addition of audible alarms on pulse oximetry and capnography [8]. The intention of standards is to codify and institutionalize specific practices that constitute safety monitoring as a strategy to prevent anesthesia accidents. The ASA is nationally recognized as a leader among medical specialty societies in the development of standards to improve patient safety. Additional ASA standards, guidelines (recommendations), consensus statements, and practice advisories have been developed. The AANA has also promoted patient safety efforts to its members through the development and publication of standards.

Closed claim project

In the mid-1980s amid professional liability insurance premium concerns, the ASA initiated the Closed Claims Study, which continues today as an ongoing project to yield important information through study of anesthesia mishaps [8]. Begun by the ASA Committee on Professional Liability, the Closed Claims Project is a standardized collection of malpractice claims against anesthesiologists. The claims are obtained from more than 30 professional liability insurance carriers and the claims (to date about 5000) for the project are reviewed by anesthesiologists who volunteer their time. The goal of the Closed Claims project is to discover unappreciated patterns of anesthesia care that may contribute to patient injury and subsequent litigation. This goal is based on the philosophy that prevention of adverse outcomes is the best method for controlling the costs of professional liability insurance. Findings from the Closed Claims Project have been published in more than 20 peer-reviewed articles.

In the late 1980s, analysis of the claims in the database revealed that respiratory-related events were the most often cited source of anesthesia liability. The reviewers also determined that most of these events could have been prevented if there had been better monitoring. These findings compelled the ASA to develop standards and guidelines relating to pulse oximetry, capnography, and management of the difficult airway. Other important studies from project data address sudden cardiac arrest during spinal anesthesia, burns from warming devices, peripheral nerve injury, intra-operative awareness, injuries from gas delivery equipment, and the effects of bias and perceived outcome on expert review of the anesthetic event.

Improved education

Improved anesthesia patient safety is thought to be in part because of the high quality of trainees who enter anesthesia residency training and the extension of the residency requirement from 2 to 3 years of clinical anesthesia after a year of general medical postgraduate training. The explosion of anesthesia textbooks, journals, and scientific and educational meetings, has contributed to the knowledge base. Sessions on patient safety topics have been incorporated into the scientific program of the ASA Annual Meeting, which has raised awareness.

Safety research

APSF awards research grants for projects that study patient safety related issues [9]. When the first APSF grants were awarded in 1987, funds for patient safety research in anesthesia were nonexistent. Since 1987, APSF has awarded more than 60 grants that total more than $2.7 million and have resulted in more than 200 publications. Among the important research topics have been patient simulation, human factors, affect of fatigue on performance, outcome assessment, and formation of carbon monoxide in the anesthesia breathing circuit.

The most important outcome of the grant awards may not be the knowledge created and disseminated, but rather the new cadre of investigators and scholars the grants have helped to develop by providing a funding source and an intellectual home for individuals who devote their careers to patient safety [1].

Simulation

In the late 1980s, supported by APSF grant funding, realistic patient simulators were introduced into anesthesiology [1,9]. Anesthesiology became the leader in the application and adoption of simulators which provide strong patient safety implications through education (resident learning new skills for the first time on a mannequin), training (teamwork, critical event management) and research (human performance). Use of realistic simulators has now become common in other medical specialties.

Present and future anesthesia patient safety initiatives

Office-based anesthesia and surgery

APSF has advocated for a single safety standard for surgical and anesthetic procedures regardless of whether these occur in the hospital, ambulatory surgical unit, or physician's office [11]. The default assumption is that a unified standard will require functionally equivalent organizational features that include equipment, staff, emergency backup, and accreditation in each of the practice locations [1]. The burden of proof to overturn this assumption rests with those who believe that the physician's office can be a safe site for anesthesia and surgery without these features.

Automated information systems

According to the APSF, the use of automated information management systems could improve the future ability to link intra-operative events to both short-term and long-term outcomes [12]. Collection of real-time, data obtained from the millions of anesthetics administered annually worldwide could lead to a better understanding of best anesthesia practices and improved patient safety. The Data Dictionary Task Force, under the sponsorship of APSF, has developed standard anesthesia terms for use in automated information systems [13]. These terms will be integrated into the Systematized Nomenclature of Medicine's core content and will be available through the National Library of Medicine.

High reliability organization theory

High Reliability Organizational (HRO) theory has many applications for the operating room environment and perioperative care [14]. An HRO organization accomplishes its mission and avoids catastrophic events, despite significant hazards, dynamic tasks, time constraints, and complex technologies. If HRO concepts are applied to the practice of anesthesiology and the perioperative period for all those who participate as part of the patient care team, anesthesia patient safety may be improved.

Audible information signals

Monitoring the patient's physiologic function during anesthesia and surgery is intended to facilitate, but not replace, the vigilance of the anesthesia profes-sional. In this regard, monitors add an additional safety net to the constant vigilance during patient care. APSF endorses use of audible alarms on physio-logic monitors despite the fact that evidence to support their value will probably never be available [3,14]. An audible tone for the pulse tone and oxygen saturation, as well as an audible tone for capnography alarm limits, is advocated by APSF as a method to enhance patient safety.

Surgical contributions to patient safety

The division of this article into a part on anesthesia and a part on surgery is arbitrary, and intended only for convenience of the authors. It does not imply a separation in the anesthesiologist's and the surgeon's respective care of the surgical patient. Jointly, anesthesiologists and surgeons are part of an integral multi-disciplinary team of providers who contribute to an overall system of care, the quality of which is the most important determinant of patient outcome in surgery.

Patient safety in surgery

In general, surgeons have perceived patient safety as safety from preventable errors. These errors have included, in part, surgery on the wrong site or side, retained foreign materials, transfusion mismatch, medication errors, mishaps in the operating room, and accidents in care, in and out of the operating room. The 1999 Institute of Medicine (IOM) report focused attention on these types of errors and cast patient safety in terms of safety from iatrogenic injury [2]. Con-sidered by some to be the most influential health care publication in two decades [15], this publication created a major national concern about patient safety and prompted a wide variety of constituencies in health care to conduct research and engage in efforts to improve patient safety. The IOM report set a goal of 50% reduction in error-related deaths over 5 years. Although there might not yet be evidence to suggest that national efforts have resulted in an overall reduction in error-related deaths [16], laudable efforts have been expended in anesthesia and surgery to achieve this goal. The Department of Veterans Affairs, through its Center for Patient Safety, has developed very specific guidelines to avoid surgery on the wrong patient, wrong site, and wrong side [17], and has mandated a time before any surgical incision, wherein the whole surgical team is briefed on the details of the intended surgical plan. The recent patient safety literature has been replete with articles and studies by surgical teams that have underscored the importance of a systems approach and proper communication to improve the safety of the operating room environment [18–21], most of which emphasize the importance of communication on patient safety. The American College of Surgeons, much like the Anesthesia Patient Safety Foundation, has also expended renewed efforts to improve patient safety in surgery. One result of these efforts is a publication by the American College of Surgeons [22] which provides a concise exposition of the state of patient safety in surgery, and is probably the best single resource for readers who want to learn more about the current conceptual framework of surgeons, and the clinical guidelines they advocate for safety of the surgical patient.

The development of the National Surgical Quality Improvement Program (NSQIP), first in the VA [23] and then in the private sector (www.acsnsqip.org) has provided the surgeons with new tools to assess and improve the quality of surgical care. A 15-year experience with the NSQIP has thrown new light on patient safety in surgery and prompts the surgical community to view patient safety in surgery in a different conceptual framework, a full understanding of which requires an understanding of the NSQIP and its achievements to date.

The National Surgical Quality Improvement Program

The NSQIP is a validated state-of-the-art system for the comparative measurement and continuous improvement of the quality of major surgery nationwide [23–25]. The comparative metric used is risk-adjusted outcome, which focuses initially on risk-adjusted 30-day morbidity and mortality. Structures, process, and cost of health care are featured as they relate to risk-adjusted outcome. Continuous improvement is achieved through feedback to providers of comparative data that include patient risk factors and risk-adjusted outcomes.

The program originated in the Veterans Health Administration and was prompted by a 1987 congressional mandate that had been issued because of concern about perceived poor outcomes of surgery in the Veterans Administration (VA). It was initiated in 1994 after the conclusion of a large observational VA study that validated the use of risk-adjusted outcomes as measures of quality of surgical care [26–28]. The program applies to outcome-based quality measurement, the same scientific rigor that is normally applied to fundamental research. A trained, dedicated clinical nurse reviewer at each medical center collects prospectively pre-operative, intra-operative, and 30-day outcome variables on most patients who undergo major surgery. Data collection methodology is standardized and nurse competency and inter-rater reliability are periodically ascertained through site visits, a web-based competency assessment program, and annual meetings of all the clinical nurse reviewers. Data are transmitted from each medical center to a national data coordination center where they are cleaned and subjected to statistical analyses. Annually, these analyses identify the independent predictors of various 30-day outcomes for all operations in a hospital, and for the various surgical subspecialties, by calculating a Beta coefficient for each predictive variable in a respective model. This coefficient is then used to calculate the expected 30-day outcome for a patient, or for a specific population of patients, based on the severity of illness of that patient or population. The ratio of the observed to the expected outcome (O/E ratio), is the risk- adjusted metric for that outcome, which is used by the NSQIP to compare the performance of the participating institutions [24]. The NSQIP has validated its O/E ratios for morbidity and mortality as reliable measures of quality within its institutions, based on an extensive site visit study [28].

Feedback of comparative data

The NSQIP provides an outcome-based comparative measure of quality of surgical centers, and affects quality improvement through extensive feedback to the providers of comparative preoperative and risk-adjusted outcome data, which are used locally to drive and monitor process improvement [29]. Significant reductions in morbidity and mortality O/E ratios, as a result of local quality improvement efforts at various surgical centers, are repeatedly observed in the NSQIP [25]. In the decade after the inception of the NSQIP, the 30-day mortality rate in the VA following major surgery has decreased by 31% and the 30-day post-operative morbidity rate has decreased by 45%. A 2002 Institute of Medicine report cited the VA Health System as "best in the nation" in part because of NSQIP, which it referred to as "one of the most highly regarded VHA initiatives employing performance measures" [30].

Quality improvement through observational studies

The NSQIP effects quality improvement through feedback to providers of comparative data, but also seeks to provide an infrastructure for its surgical investigators to conduct hypothesis-driven outcome studies using its rich clinical database, which contains full clinical and outcome data on nearly 1.4 million major operations. To date, more than 75 papers emanating from the NSQIP have been published in peer-reviewed journals. The subjects of these studies have varied over a wide range of topics which included predictive models for specific outcomes and complications, racial and other variations in outcomes of surgical care, appropriateness of treatment for a variety of specific surgical conditions, the volume outcome relationship, and more. A full list of these publications is available on the website of the American College of Surgeons (www.acsnsqip.org). Two recently completed studies that were the result of collaboration between the NSQIP and the American College of Surgeons are The Patient Safety in Surgery Study, and the Working Conditions Study. The results of these studies are currently being analyzed to determine the relationship to outcomes of specific in-hospital processes and provider conditions that are thought to relate to patient and environmental safety. Cumulatively, the publications and studies of the NSQIP provide information that promote patient safety not only by enabling the linkage of patient safety processes to patient outcomes, but also by promoting quality improvement through a reduction in postoperative morbidity and mortality rates, that is, contributing to a safer domain within a system of surgical care.

The private sector

To ascertain the applicability of the NSQIP to the private sector, the NSQIP started its Private Sector Initiative (PSI) in 1998. Three academic non-VA surgical departments volunteered to provide a full-time nurse and to participate in the NSQIP in a manner identical to the VA hospitals. A special web-based system for the collection of data from these three sites and for their transmission to the VA data coordination and analysis center was created. Data in the PSI were limited to general and vascular surgery. Analysis of the first year of data collected from the three alpha sites (Emory University Hospital, Atlanta; University of Kentucky Medical Center, Lexington; and University of Michigan Medical Center, Ann Arbor) showed that the processes, methodology, and 30-day outcome predictive models, developed by the VA NSQIP, were fully applicable to the private sector, at least in general and vascular surgery [5]. Based on this result, the VA and the American College of Surgeons collaborated together to apply for, and ultimately conduct, the Patient Safety in Surgery (PSS) Study, which was funded by the Agency for Health Care Research and Quality. Also limited to general and vascular surgery, this study included participation in the NSQIP by 14 non-VA large academic medical centers and 4 smaller community hospitals (ie, 18 Beta sites) over a 3-year data collection period which terminated on September 30, 2004. The results of this study are currently being prepared for publication. The study met its objectives and demonstrated that the NSQIP was equally applicable to private sector hospitals as to the VA hospitals. The methodology could be easily implemented in the private sector, the predictive models were similar, and the variation in risk-adjusted outcomes was equally as wide, which reflected similar variation in quality of surgical care. As in the VA, application of the NSQIP to the private sector prompted local quality improvement initiatives that resulted in improvement of outcomes in those facilities. As stated above, data from the PSS Study is currently being analyzed to determine the linkage between structures and processes of care that are thought to be related to patient safety and patient outcomes.

The results of the PSS study prompted the American College of Surgeons, in late 1994, to establish the ACS-NSQIP that uses methodology, process, and structure identical to those of the VA NSQIP. Initially, however, the ACS-NSQIP has enrolled only patients who undergo general or vascular surgery. To date, more than 60 private hospitals are enrolled in the ACS-NSQIP, and approximately 80 have completed their applications to join. Details of the program can be found on the ACS website (www.acsnsqip.org).

What have we learned?

The experience gained from the operational aspect of the NSQIP in both the VA and the private sector, and the knowledge gained from the numerous observational studies that have emanated from its database, prompt us to view patient safety in a totally different framework from the one that was popularized by the IOM report [2]. This view is based on three important patient-safety-related observations made by the NSQIP:

> 1. Safety is indistinguishable from overall quality of surgical care and should not be addressed independent of surgical quality.

The wide variation in the morbidity and mortality O/E ratios among various institutions, and the demonstrated ability of local process improvement to significantly lower these ratios, clearly indicate that, during an episode of surgical care, certain populations of patients are safer than others. After all, all morbidity is injurious to the patient and mortality is the ultimate lack of patient safety. Regardless of whether it is preventable or not, an adverse outcome compromises patient safety. The NSQIP has demonstrated, through its day-to-day operation and in several observational studies, that rates of adverse outcomes, properly measured and risk-adjusted, can reflect the quality of surgical care. If patient safety is placed within the rubric of quality and defined in terms of safety from adverse outcomes, we can use the same quantitative tools that the NSQIP has developed for assessment and improvement of quality, to assess and improve patient safety. Improved quality of surgical care reduces the incidence of adverse outcomes and improves patient safety. Within this rubric, prevention of errors is synonymous with reduction of adverse outcomes, and, as such, can be a reliable quality measure.

> 2. During an episode of surgical care, adverse outcomes, and hence patient safety, are primarily determined by quality of *systems* of care.

Several times in the course of a year, the NSQIP is asked to visit surgical departments that have significantly higher than expected O/E ratios in mortality or morbidity. An experienced team of a surgeon, a nurse, and an anesthesiologist conduct the site visit in accordance with a structured instrument that evaluates the structures and processes of care at the hospital. Invariably, structures or processes are found to be problematic at high-outlier hospitals, which reflect deficiencies in systems of care. Errors in these hospitals, although sometimes committed by specific providers, are more likely to be system errors rather than provider incompetence. The provider is important in as much as he or she contributes to the system. These site visits have underscored the importance of adequate communication, coordination, and team work to achieve quality surgical care, which confirms publications from the National Surgical Risk Study that had addressed these issues [31,32].

> 3. Reliable comparative outcome data are imperative for the identification of system problems and the assurance of patient safety from adverse outcomes.

Surgeons in the VA have learned that although obvious iatrogenic and accidental provider errors can be easily detected through good local quality monitoring systems, the more subtle system errors that lead to a much larger body of adverse outcomes cannot be adequately appreciated or recognized without comparative data with other institutions and peer groups [29]. Deficiencies and errors within a system of care can result in adverse outcome rates that might be considered acceptable by the local provider community, particularly when comparisons are made with unadjusted rates published in the literature. It is only when these rates are compared with similarly risk-adjusted rates at other peer institutions that the providers appreciate the increased adversity at their center, and are thus prompted to investigate and improve the quality of the adversity-related processes and structures.

Fig. 1 represents a conceptual framework for patient safety in anesthesia and surgery which takes into account the lessons learned from the NSQIP. Within every system of care for the surgical patient, there is an unsafe domain that comprises the totality of the adverse outcomes experienced by patients who are cared for within that system. Preventable errors form a very small part of the unsafe domain, which is dominated by the usual adverse postoperative complications and outcomes. Sentinel events are also not the only preventable adverse outcomes within the system. Preventability is represented in Fig. 1 by a spectrum with white on one end, which represents preventable adverse outcomes, and black on the other, which represents unpreventable adverse outcomes. Potentially, every adverse outcome should be preventable when quality improvement efforts intensify within a system of care and the size of the unsafe domain is reduced: the better the quality of care, the less the adverse outcomes, and the smaller the unsafe domain. Hence, the size of the unsafe domain is a good measure of quality of care, makes safety and quality one and the same. In a quality and safe system of surgical care (statistically low-outlier by NSQIP criteria), the size of the unsafe

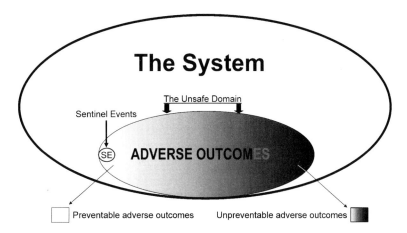

Fig. 1. A conceptual schema which illustrates patient safety in surgery is inseparable from quality of surgical care. Within a surgical system of care there is an unsafe domain, which comprises the totality of the adverse outcomes experienced by patients who are cared for by the system. Within this domain, the adverse outcomes vary over a spectrum of preventability. Sentinel events, which have been the focus of numerous national patient safety initiatives, are preventable errors that comprise a very small fraction of the unsafe domain. Local quality improvement initiatives that reduce the incidence of preventable adverse outcomes should reduce the size of the unsafe domain and, within it, the ratio of preventable to unpreventable adverse outcomes.

domain would be small and the ratio of preventable to unpreventable adverse outcomes would also be small. Conversely, in a poor and unsafe system of surgical care (statistically high-outlier by NSQIP criteria), the size of the unsafe domain would be large as would be the ratio of preventable to unpreventable adverse outcomes. One can appreciate from this construct that it would be futile to address patient safety only in terms of sentinel events, and the error one would commit by excluding system errors from the definition of patient safety, which account for most of the preventable adverse postoperative outcomes.

The IOM report called for the institution of national efforts and initiatives that would reduce the incidence of preventable errors by 50%. Although the report prompted an avalanche of new national initiatives, undertaken by various governmental and non-governmental constituencies to enhance patient safety, 6 years later there is no clear evidence that these types of errors have been substantially reduced at the national level [16]. In light of the conceptual construct of safety described above, the failure to reduce the incidence of iatrogenic errors over 5 years (or at least the uncertainty about it), may be because of (1) the ipso facto separation in the IOM report of accidental and preventable errors from the wider domain of adverse outcomes, (2) the wrong assumption that most preventable errors are readily recognizable, and (3) misdirection of the safety focus to individual provider errors that might lead to an increase in the incidence of sentinel events, rather than direction of the focus to system errors that are difficult to recognize and that might lead to increased incidence of much more frequent adverse postoperative outcomes. An unmistakably preventable provider error can still be a reflection of system error. If engineered properly, a quality system of care with proper checks and balances should prevent provider vulnerability from making an error in as much as it should prevent patient vulnerability from developing an adverse intra- or post-operative outcome. Focusing on preventable iatrogenic injury caused by the provider and quantified by the rate of sentinel events, ignores the much larger domain of preventable iatrogenic patient injury caused by the system and quantified by the risk-adjusted rate of adverse outcomes.

Long-term patient safety

Most efforts to improve anesthesia patient safety to date have been focused on adverse events in the immediate perioperative period. Over the last few years, several threads of information (eg, protective effect of beta-adrenergic blockers against subsequent myocardial infarction) have coalesced and suggest anesthesia and surgery may influence adverse outcomes that occur remote from the perioperative period (ie, well beyond the first 30 postoperative days) [33–36]. Intra-operative management by both anesthesiologists and surgeons may have profound effects on long-term patient outcomes. This effect has probably not been adequately appreciated because of limitations in both monitoring technologies and information transfer infrastructure in the operating room. In a well-conducted observational study of 1064 patients who underwent general anesthesia, Monk and colleagues [35] identified three independent predictors of 1-year post-operative mortality: the compendium of patient comorbidity, cumulative deep hypnotic time as quantified by Bisectral Index < 45, and intra-operative systolic hypotension. The study underscores an important paradigm: intra-operative management may affect outcomes over longer time periods than previously appreciated. Although not well established, the study lends credence to the possibility that anesthetic drugs, other aspects of the anesthetic technique, or physiologic occurrences during surgery could be potent triggers for abnormal inflammation. Although contested by some [37–39], depth of anesthesia may be an important consideration and perhaps act as a marker for patients who have a different (perhaps genetically determined) physiologic state which manifests as enhanced autonomic nervous system activity [35]. These individuals might be more likely to be treated with higher levels of hypnotics or volatile anesthetics based on clinical signs during anesthesia.

Another recent study that established a relationship between intra-operative management and long-term outcomes involved 496 patients who underwent cardiac surgery on cardiopulmonary bypass and who were followed-up for an average of 10 years postoperatively [36]. In these patients, intra-myocardial tissue pH, a reliable measure of regional myocardial ischemia, was monitored in the anterior and posterior walls of the left ventricle throughout the duration of open median sternotomy. Specific levels of myocardial tissue acidosis observed before, during, and after the period of aortic clamping were shown to be independent determinants of long-term survival. For example, the median survival of patients who experienced a mean myocardial pH $\leq$ 6.34 during the period of aortic clamping was independently reduced by 34% compared with patients who experienced a mean myocardial pH > 6.34 during this period (Fig. 2). Basic studies by the same group of investigators had shown that myocardial acidosis of this magnitude was a primary trigger of myocyte apoptosis [40], but the relationships of the latter to late congestive heart failure, or to the inflammatory and immunologic responses, remain unknown.

To date, the most dramatic evidence of a link between in-hospital events and long- term outcomes comes from an NSQIP study that was recently presented to the American Surgical Association in its last annual meeting [41]. The purpose of the study was to identify variables in an episode of surgical care that were independent determinants of long-term survival after major surgery. Records in the NSQIP database of 105,951 patients who underwent 8 types of major surgery were merged with the Veterans Benefits Administration database, the BIRLS file, which has proven to be 87%–95% accurate for depicting the vital status of US veterans. The study showed that over a mean follow-up period of 8 years, the most important determinant of decreased post-operative survival was the occurrence, within 30 days postoperatively, of any one of 22 types of complications collected in the NSQIP. Independent of preoperative patient risk, the occurrence of a 30-day complication in the total patient group reduced median patient survival by 69%, a wound complication reduced the median survival by 42%, and

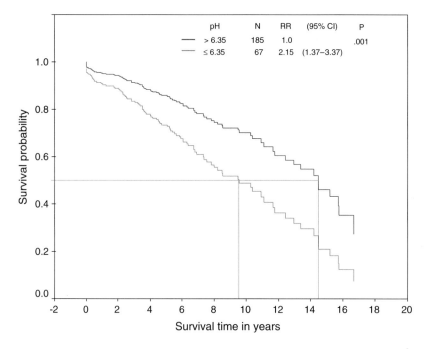

Fig. 2. Survival probability curves (adjusted for other variables in Cox proportional hazards regression model: age, preoperative ejection fraction, diabetes, year of surgery, operation type, surgeon, cardioplegia type, duration of aortic clamping, and duration of cardiopulmonary bypass) of patients who underwent cardiac surgery and in whom mean myocardial pH (corrected to 37 degrees centigrade = pH_{37C}) during aortic clamping was > 6.34 (*top line*) and patients in whom it was ≤ 6.34 (*bottom line*). Risk ratio (RR) and 95% confidence interval (CI) of the group with lower pH_{37C} versus the group with higher pH_{37C} are shown. The vertical line at 50% survival probability defines median survival for each patient group. After accounting for all other confounding variables, patients who experienced acidosis with pH_{37c} below threshold in either the anterior or the posterior left ventricular wall experienced a 34% reduction in median survival. (*From* Khuri SF, Healey NA, Hossain M, et al. Intra-operative regional myocardial acidosis and reduction in long-term survival after cardiac surgery. J Thorac Cardiovasc Surg 2005;129(2):378; with permission. © 2005 by The American Association for Thoracic Surgery.)

a pulmonary complication reduced median survival by 87%. The adverse effect of a complication on patient survival was also influenced by the operation type, and was sustained even when patients who did not survive for 30 days were excluded from the analyses (Fig. 3).

Within the broader construct of safety from adverse outcomes, there is mounting evidence that in-hospital and intra-operative management of patients by anesthesiologists and surgeons can markedly influence the long-term safety of these patients, although the underlying mechanisms for these relationships are poorly understood. As suggested above, the perioperative inflammatory and immune response may be a potential biological link to long-term outcomes after anesthesia and surgery [33,34]. It is conceivable that the inflammatory response

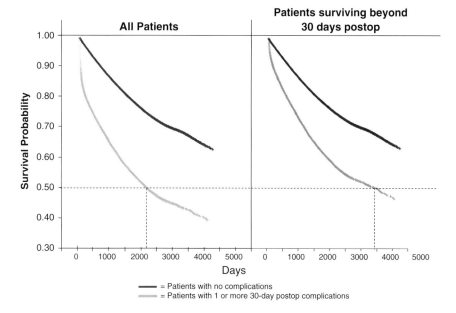

Fig. 3. (*Left*) Cox survival curves of all study patients who sustained a 30-day postoperative complication compared with those who did not. (*Right*) Cox survival curves of study patients who survived 30 days after major surgery stratified as to whether or not patients had sustained a complication within the first 30 postoperative days. The difference in survival between the two groups in each panel reflects the independent effect of the occurrence of a postoperative complication on postoperative survival, corrected for other confounding variables captured in the NSQIP database. (*From* Khuri SF, Henderson WG, DePalma RG, et al. Determinants of long-term survival after major surgery and the adverse effect of postoperative complications. Ann Surg 2005;242(3):334; with permission.)

to surgery may amplify proinflammatory cell mechanisms of certain disease states, such as coronary artery disease, and hence contribute to disease acceleration and adverse perioperative events. It is possible that certain patients or patient populations may exhibit an exaggerated inflammatory response to surgery or delayed resolution of the preoperative immune status. If true, these patients may be at even greater risk for postoperative complications. Inflammatory processes, and complications that exaggerate them may accelerate apoptosis in a manner similar to the well-known effect of acidosis on apoptosis [40]. An APSF task-force is evaluating available data in order to recommend future strategies for the study of perioperative factors that might influence long-term outcomes. One such strategy, which is currently pursued by both APSF and NSQIP, is the development of an information technology (IT) infrastructure that would make it possible to merge data obtained for intra-operative automated information systems, with patient risk and outcome data obtained from the NSQIP. Efforts like this will lead to better understanding of the linkage between intra-operative events and patient outcomes.

Summary

In their care of a surgical patient, the anesthesiologist and the surgeon are part of a single team that functions within a unified system of care, the quality of which is a major determinant of patient outcome. Reference to outcome of anesthesia versus outcome of surgery is purely arbitrary, because the ultimate outcome is that of the patient, and that outcome is influenced by the totality of the providers involved in the patient's care.

Anesthesiology has served as a model for patient safety in health care and was the first medical profession to treat patient safety as an independent problem. Anesthesiology has implemented widely accepted guidelines on basic monitoring, conducted long-term analyses of closed malpractice claims, developed patient simulators as meaningful training tools, and addressed problems of human error. Most importantly the profession has institutionalized safety through the creation of the ASA Committee on Patient Safety and Risk Management and the Anesthesia Patient Safety Foundation. Financial support of patient safety investigations has resulted in meaningful safety research as well as the creation of a cadre of safety investigators for the future.

As in aviation, many of the accepted and proposed safety changes in anesthesia lack evidence-based support, but the common theme is they make sense and are the right thing to do (monitoring standards, audible information signals, HRO theory, automated information systems). Evidence from randomized trials is important but it is neither sufficient nor necessary for acceptance of safety practices [3]. There will never be complete evidence for everything that needs to be done in medicine. The prudent alternative is to make reasonable judgments based on the best available evidence. The perceived decrease in anesthesia morbidity and mortality over the last 20 years is not attributable to any single practice or development of new anesthetic drugs, but rather to application of a broad array of changes in process, equipment, organization, supervision, training, and teamwork [3]. No one of these changes has ever been proven to have a clear-cut impact on mortality. Rather, anesthesia safety was achieved through the application of a host of changes that made sense; were based on sound principles, technical theory, or experience; and addressed real-life clinical issues. Anesthesiology showed that safety is doing a lot of little things that, in the aggregate, make a big difference [3].

Despite improvements in anesthesia patient safety, opportunity for further advances in safety remains. Anesthesia is not yet completely safe, even for otherwise healthy patients whose greatest risk may be iatrogenic and systems-related complications [5]. Anesthesiologists must remain motivated to continue to pursue harmless anesthesia, yet at the same time be proud leaders of patient safety [6].

Experience with the National Surgical Quality Improvement Program to date, prompts us to place patient safety in anesthesia and surgery within a much larger conceptual framework than that of safety from preventable iatrogenic injury and sentinel events. The NSQIP, which was developed in the Department of Veterans Affairs and has been recently extended to the private sector through the American

College of Surgeons, is the first national, validated, and peer-controlled program that uses risk-adjusted outcomes for the comparative assessment and improvement of the quality of surgical care. The program has reduced postoperative complications in the VA, both nationally and at the local level, in individual VA medical centers. The NSQIP experience prompts the redefinition of patient safety in terms of safety from all adverse postoperative outcomes, and supports three important paradigms related to patient safety in anesthesia and surgery:

1. Safety is indistinguishable from overall quality of surgical care and should not be addressed independent of surgical quality.

Efforts currently expended on patient safety should not be separate from efforts expended on improving quality.

2. During an episode of surgical care, adverse outcomes, and hence patient safety, are primarily determined by the quality of care systems.

The anesthesiologist and surgeon are important in as much as he or she contributes to the quality of the system.

3. Reliable comparative outcome data are imperative for the identification of system problems and the ultimate assurance of patient safety from adverse outcomes.

It is becoming more evident that processes and events that occur during surgery can be important determinants of long-term outcomes after anesthesia and surgery. Inflammatory and immune processes precipitated by the surgical insult and by early postoperative adverse outcomes might help determine this relationship. Therefore, efforts should be expended to improve patient safety in the long term by: (1) gaining a better understanding of the impact of specific events on the inflammatory and immune systems, and (2) enhancing the IT infrastructure to facilitate acquisition of important intra-operative data and linking these data to the clinical short- and long-term outcomes of these patients.

Acknowledgments

The authors acknowledge with gratitude the editorial help of Nancy Healey.

References

[1] Gaba DM. Anaesthesiology as a model for patient safety in health care. BMJ 2000;320:785–8.
[2] Kohn L, Corrigan J, Donaldson M, editors. To err is human: building a safer health care system. Washington: National Academy Press; 2000. Available at: http://darwin.nap.edu/books/0309068371/html/.

[3] Leape LL, Berwick DM, Bates DW. What practices will most improve safety? Evidence-based medicine meets patient safety. JAMA 2002;288:501–7.

[4] Eichhorn JH. Prevention of intraoperative anesthesia accidents and related severe injury through safety monitoring. Anesthesiology 1989;70:572–7.

[5] Lagasse RS. Anesthesia safety: model or myth? A review of the published literature and analysis of current original data. Anesthesiology 2002;97:1609–17.

[6] Cooper JB, Gaba D. No myth: anesthesia is a model for addressing patient safety. Anesthesiology 2002;97:1335–7.

[7] Tomlin J. The deep sleep: 6,000 will die or suffer brain damage [transcript]. 20/20. WLS-TV. April 22, 1982.

[8] Pierce EC. The 34th Rovenstine lecture: 40 years behind the mask: safety revisited. Anesthesiology 1996;84:965–75.

[9] Stoelting RK. A historical review of the origin and contributions of the Anesthesia Patient Safety Foundation. ASA 100 Newsletter (Special Commemorative Issue 1905–2005) 2005. Available at: www.asahq.org/newsletters/2005/centennial/szabat100.html.

[10] Cooper JB, Newbower RS, Long CD, et al. Preventable anesthesia mishaps: a study of human factors. Anesthesiology 1978;49:399–406.

[11] Stoelting RK. Office-based anesthesia growth provokes safety fears. APSF Newlsetter (Spring) 2000;15(1). Available at: www.apsf.org/resource_center/newsletters.mspx.

[12] Gravenstein NS. Information systems: new role of information in anesthesia patient safety highlighted in a series of articles by technology experts. APSF Newsletter (Summer) 2001;16(2). Available at: www.apsf.org/resource_center/newsletters.mspx.

[13] Stoelting RK. Data dictionary task force (DDTF) launches initiative. APSF Newlsetter (Summer) 2002;17(2).

[14] Gaba DM. Safety first: ensuring quality are in the intensely productive environment-the HRO model. APSF Newsletter (Spring) 2003;18(1).

[15] Altman DE, Clancy C, Blendon RJ. Improving patient safety five years after the IOM report. N Engl J Med 2004;351:2041–3.

[16] Brennan TA, Gawande A, Thomas E, et al. Accidental deaths, saved lives, and improved quality. N Engl J Med 2005;353(13):1405–9.

[17] Department of Veterans Affairs National Center for Patient Safety. Frequent questions on marking the surgical site. OR Manager 2003;19(2):18–9.

[18] Vincent C, Moorthy K, Sarker SK, et al. Systems approaches to surgical quality and safety: from concept to measurement. Ann Surg 2004;239(4):475–82.

[19] Awad SS, Fagan SP, Bellows C, et al. Bridging the communication gap in the operating room with medical team training. Am J Surg 2005;190(5):770–4.

[20] Lingard L, Espin S, Whyte S, et al. Communication failures in the operating room: an observational classification of recurrent types and effects. Qual Saf Health Care 2004;13(5):330–4.

[21] Lingard L, Espin S, Rubin B, et al. Getting teams to talk: development and pilot implementation of a checklist to promote interprofessional communication in the OR. Qual Saf Health Care 2005;14(5):340–6.

[22] Manuel BM, Nora PF, editors. Surgical patient safety: essential information for surgeons in today's environment. Chicago: American College of Surgeons; 2004.

[23] Khuri SF, Daley J, Henderson W, et al. The Department of Veteran's Affairs NSQIP: the first national validated, outcome-based, risk-adjusted, and peer-controlled program for the measurement and enhancement of the quality of surgical care. Ann Surg 1998;228(4):491–507.

[24] Khuri S, Daley J, Henderson WG. The comparative assessment and improvement of quality of surgical care in the Department of Veterans Affairs. Arch Surg 2002;137(1):20–7.

[25] Khuri SF. The NSQIP: a new frontier in surgery. Surgery 2005;138(5):19–25.

[26] Khuri SF, Daley J, Henderson W, et al. Risk adjustment of the postoperative mortality rate for the comparative assessment of the quality of surgical care. Results of the National VA Surgical Risk Study. J Am Coll Surg 1997;185(4):315–27.

[27] Daley J, Khuri SF, Henderson W, et al. Risk adjustment of the postoperative morbidity rate for the comparative assessment of the quality of surgical care. Results of the National VA Surgical Risk Study. J Am Coll Surg 1997;185(4):328–40.

[28] Daley J, Forbes MG, Young GJ, et al. Validating risk-adjusted surgical outcomes: site visit assessment of process and structure. J Am Coll Surg 1997;185(4):341–51.

[29] Neumayer L, Mastin M, Vanderhoof L, et al. Using the Veterans Administration National Surgical Quality Improvement Program to improve patient outcomes. J Surg Res 2000;88:58–61.

[30] Hewett M. Interpreting the volume-outcome relationship in the context of health care quality. Workshop summary. Institute of Medicine. Washington: National Academies Press; 2000.

[31] Young GJ, Charns MP, Daley J. Best practices for managing surgical services: the role of coordination. J Healthcare Management Rev 1997;22(4):85–99.

[32] Young GJ, Charns MP, Desai K, et al. Patterns of coordination and clinical outcomes: a study of surgical services. Health Serv Res 1998;33:1211–36.

[33] Meiler SE, Monk TG, Mayfield JB, et al. Can we alter long-term outcome? The role of anesthetic management and the inflammatory responses. APSF Newsletter (Fall) 2003;18(3).

[34] Meiler SE, Monk TG, Mayfield JB, et al. Can we alter long-term outcome? The role of inflammation and immunity in the perioperative period (Part II). APSF Newsletter (Spring) 2004;19(1).

[35] Monk TG, Saini V, Weldon BC, et al. Anesthetic management and one-year mortality after noncardiac surgery. Anesth Analg 2005;100:4–10.

[36] Khuri SF, Healey NA, Hossain M, et al. Intra-operative regional myocardial acidosis and reduction in long-term survival after cardiac surgery. J Thorac Cardiovasc Surg 2005;192(2):372–81.

[37] Levy WJ. Is anesthetic-related mortality a statistical illness? [letter]. Anesth Analg 2005;101:1238.

[38] Berry AJ. Observational studies identify associations, not causality [letter]. Anesth Analg 2005;101:1238.

[39] Drummond JC. Editorial board reproached for publication of BIS-mortality correlation [letter]. Anesth Analg 2005;101:1238–9.

[40] Thatte HS, Rhee JH, Zagarins S, et al. Acidosis induced apoptosis in the human and porcine heart. Ann Thorac Surg 2004;77:1376–83.

[41] Khuri SF, Henderson WG, DePalma RG, et al. Determinants of long-term survival after major surgery and the adverse effect of postoperative complications. Ann Surg 2005;242(3):326–43.

ELSEVIER
SAUNDERS

Anesthesiology Clin N Am
24 (2006) 255–278

ANESTHESIOLOGY
CLINICS OF
NORTH AMERICA

Long-term Outcome After Anesthesia and Surgery: Remarks on the Biology of a Newly Emerging Principle in Perioperative Care

Steffen E. Meiler, MD

*Program of Molecular Perioperative Medicine & Genomics,
Department of Anesthesiology and Perioperative Medicine, Medical College of Georgia,
1150 15th Street, BIW 2144, Augusta, GA 30912-2700, USA*

Although there is risk in writing about a subject in the absence of a solid scientific or experiential foundation, science cannot always operate within safe confines. Sometimes risk must be assumed, especially when a finding seems capable of opening up broad new avenues of research and patient care. One such finding is the emerging epidemiologic evidence of a possible link between the variables of the perioperative process and long-term risk after surgery. The potential significance of this link to long-term risk led the Anesthesia Patient Safety Foundation (APSF)—in a radical departure from its traditional focus on risk reduction in the immediate perioperative period—to convene a panel of experts from multiple medical specialties and government and health quality organizations to discuss it in September 2004 [1]. The 2004 APSF panel concluded that, although evidence is sparse, anesthesia and surgery may contribute to excess morbidity and mortality months (or even years) after surgery. If confirmed the implications of this extended risk period are enormous and will challenge the health care community to amend established priorities of care delivery, patient follow-up, and research focus.

According to statistics on postoperative mortality, 5% to 14% of elderly and other high-risk groups die within 1 year after surgery [2–4]. The principal causes of death are cardiovascular disease and cancer, just as in the general population, but their incidence seems to be increased after surgery. These numbers are in stark contrast to the much lower mortality that is seen in the weeks immediately

E-mail address: smeiler@mcg.edu

0889-8537/06/$ – see front matter © 2006 Elsevier Inc. All rights reserved.
doi:10.1016/j.atc.2006.03.002

following surgery [5,6]. It would seem then that the stakes in perioperative care are much higher than believed previously. If, as more and more studies suggest, specific interventions in the perioperative period can reduce this long-term risk, many thousands of lives could be saved each year.

To substantiate this long-term model, its underlying biology must be elucidated. Although an arduous task, the molecular mechanisms that are responsible for this long-term influence must be deciphered if we are to develop effective therapies. Because little information on this biology is available, a broad conceptual approach will have to do for now. In the most general terms, we could hypothesize that the biologic response to the perioperative process is capable of accelerating the progression of preexisting disease states from their natural course, which results in earlier, and possibly more severe, disease-related complications. Although it is not known whether the signals that trigger this process act acutely and then fade or whether they enhance disease activity for longer periods, research into their biologic origin and functioning opens therapeutic opportunities to mitigate the long-term risks. Such opportunities do not come without challenges. The intimidatingly complex variables of the perioperative process and the patients' predictably diverse biologic responses to them make it difficult to create a rough blueprint to guide scientific activity in this endeavor.

The author is confident that such difficulties can be overcome. At the 2004 APSF Meeting, he proposed to use an immunologic model for generating and testing hypotheses as we begin to probe the biology of this postulated long-term effect [7,8]. This proposition builds on available evidence and creates a conceptual outline for clinical trials and laboratory research. An immune-based model of long-term outcome incorporates our knowledge of the profound immune-modulating effects of the perioperative experience. It considers a large body of evidence on the role of the inflammatory response on short-term outcomes and extends these insights to the biology of more remote outcome events. Beyond inflammation, it also emphasizes changes in adaptive immunity as a trigger for disease progression. Finally, one of its principal functions is to integrate this information with the staggering discoveries that are being made in the immunology of chronic disease.

One of the great lessons of modern immunology has been the realization that many of today's chronic illnesses (Box 1) originate or progress in a cellular milieu of chronic inflammation, and surprisingly, that diverse disease processes (eg, coronary artery disease, Alzheimer's disease, or some of the cancers) show significant overlap in inflammatory phenotypes [9]. Considering that anesthesia and surgery have wide-ranging effects on the immune system and incite pro-inflammatory and immunosuppressive responses [10], it seems plausible that long-term complications could originate at the interface of the perioperative immune response to the cell (and immune) mechanisms of chronic illness. Finally, this model not only assists in the selection of new candidate drugs and interventions for clinical testing, it provides additional stimulus for researching the immune response to injury and infection, places strong emphasis on genetic or acquired defects in this process, provides focus for the development of much-

Box 1. Examples of inflammatory disorders

Chronic disorders in which an important pathogenetic role is assigned to inflammation

Alzheimer's disease
Ankylosing spondylitis
Asthma
Atherosclerosis
Atopic dermatitis
Chronic obstructive pulmonary disease
Crohn's disease (regional enteritis)
Gout
Hashimoto's thyroiditis
Multiple sclerosis
Osteoarthritis
Pemphigus
Periodic fever syndromes
Psoriasis
Rheumatoid arthritis
Sarcoidosis
Systemic lupus erythematosus
Type 1 diabetes mellitus
Ulcerative colitis
Vasculitides (Wegener's syndrome, Goodpasture's syndrome, giant cell arthritis, polyarteritis nodosa)

Diseases of infectious origin in which inflammation may contribute as much to pathology as does microbial toxicity

Bacterial dysentery
Chagas disease (*Trypanosoma cruzi*)
Cystic fibrosis pneumonitis
Filariasis
Helicobacter pylori gastritis
Hepatitis C
Influenza virus pneumonia
Leprosy (tuberculoid form)
Neisserial or pneumococcal meningitis
Poststreptococcal glomerulonephritis
Sepsis syndrome
Tuberculosis

Modified from Nathan C. Points of control in inflammation. Nature 2002;420(6917):846–52.

needed animal models for research into long-term outcomes, and engages investigators who are working in several specialties—in the laboratory and in the clinic—in the common enterprise of improving patients' progress.

Perioperative variables with reported long-term effects on patient safety

Our specialty has been appreciated widely for analyzing and reducing risk factors in the immediate perioperative period and for inspiring a national effort to reduce medical errors and improve patient safety throughout our health care system [11]; however, only recently did we recognize the relationship between perioperative care and long-term risk and added it to our list of patient safety concerns. This new focus on long-term outcome affects how we care for patients, and requires that we document and study better the remote effects of perioperative events and drug use. At this point, only a handful of studies have attempted to do this, which provide only a narrow evidentiary backbone on this subject. We must examine the evidence that is available to us carefully, strive to entrench this new concept more firmly into the vernacular of our specialty, and encourage much more extensive studies.

Blood transfusions

Opelz and colleagues reported one of the earliest examples of a single perioperative intervention that changed the outcome of a remote postoperative event in 1973. In this precyclosporine era, Opelz and others found that renal allograft survival increased by ~20% after preoperative blood transfusions [12–14]. Even in studies that were conducted after the introduction of modern immunosuppressive regimens, however, Opelz and his colleagues [15] demonstrated in a prospective, multicenter study of 423 cadaver kidney recipients that pretransplant blood transfusions conferred a 9% graft survival advantage at 5 years and significantly reduced the number of rejection episodes. Many human studies have established firmly that perioperative blood transfusions provide this protection, with animal studies offering further validation. Although the exact mechanism by which allogeneic blood affords increased protection is not known, the induction of suppressor cells [16–18], the induction of mixed chimerism [18], clonal deletion [19], and the selection of low responders [20] have been proposed as possible theories. Regardless of the underlying mechanisms, it is well accepted that blood transfusions alter immune function—known as transfusion-associated immunomodulation (TRIM)—which can cause defects in cell-mediated immunity, antigen presentation, natural killer cell function, and other aspects of the immune system [21,22].

Understandably, TRIM has raised the concern that perioperative blood transfusions, although beneficial in the transplant setting, may increase the risk for surgical infections, cancer recurrence, and overall postoperative mortality. Given the findings by Khuri and colleagues (see later discussion), a transfusion-associated infection risk demands our attention because it predicts complications in the immediate days and weeks after surgery and could decrease long-term survival rates. A recent meta-analysis of 20 peer-reviewed articles that included 13,152 patients (5215 who received transfusions and 7937 who did not) evaluated the association of allogeneic (homologous) blood transfusions with the incidence of postoperative bacterial infections, with a subgroup analysis in patients who sustained trauma [23]. This report concluded that blood transfusions during or after elective surgery are associated overwhelmingly with an increased risk for postoperative infection (common odds ratio 3.45; range, 1.43–15.15), and that the risk was even greater in patients who sustained trauma (common odds ratio 5.263; range, 5.03–5.43). Other investigators have counseled that we approach these findings with reserve, because they may have been skewed by patient selection bias, observation bias, problems with blinding, and failure to provide sufficient information on the severity of illness and distribution of risk factors. Overall, however, with so many studies showing a statistically significant association, clinicians should take this evidence into account when deciding whether to transfuse; should reexamine older, more liberal transfusion guidelines; and should be aware of the modern estimate of the therapeutic benefits of transfused blood.

Furthermore, blood transfusions have been linked to another long-term outcome: the recurrence of malignancy and the progression of tumor growth after cancer surgery. According to a January 2006 Cochrane Report based on 36 studies (randomized controlled trials, prospective cohorts, and retrospective surveys), most of this research, which was conducted primarily in colorectal cancer, indicates a moderate association between perioperative transfusions and cancer recurrence risk (odds ratio [OR], 1.42; 95% CI, 1.20–1.67) [24]. Although the report does not claim a causal relationship, it concludes that carefully restricted indications for perioperative blood transfusions seem to be warranted. It remains a matter of national debate whether any of the stated risks that are associated with TRIM can be diminished with leukocyte-reduced blood transfusions [25,26].

Postoperative complications

Some of the strongest evidence to date in support of this long-term effect comes from an analysis of the National Surgical Quality Improvement Program (NSQIP) database, which contains perioperative and outcome information on more than 1.2 million major operations that were performed at Veterans' Administration hospitals nationwide over the last 15 years [27]. Specifically, this study merged the data files of NSQIP and the Beneficiary Identification and Records Locator Subsystem to identify predictors of short- ($\leq$30 days) or long-term (1 and 5 years) survival after surgery from a large number of perioperative variables. This study was based on a step-wise multiple logistic regression analysis and included data from 105,951 patients for eight different major operations over an average follow-up period of 8 years. The occurrence of any 30-day postoperative complication had a strong, independent effect on long-term survival. In patients with postoperative complications, mortality at 1 and 5 years were 28.1% and 57.6%, respectively, in contrast to 6.9% and 39.5% in patients that did not have postoperative events. Among the various types of complications that were investigated, pneumonia, deep wound infections, and myocardial infarction (MI) had some of the strongest effects on survival. This study strongly argues that adverse events after surgery can have a lasting effect on the health and life of our patients, and forces us to redefine our notion of, and temporal assumptions about, surgical risk. It is possible that the observed association between postoperative complications and mortality functions as a proxy for something else. To the extent that statistical analysis can address this issue, the investigators of this study assure us that the observed effect was independent of any other preoperative risk variable or intraoperative event. If this analysis is correct, then managing these postoperative complications successfully may not suffice to prevent their long-term effects. If we are to protect patients against such long-term effects, a thoughtful and stringently implemented hospital-wide approach is needed urgently to prevent the occurrence of early complications.

Pharmacologic interventions

β-Blockers

The last decade produced a wealth of studies that were directed at finding therapies to reduce the cardiac risk from anesthesia and surgery (see the article by Shilling and Durieux elsewhere in this issue). Among these, a few studies that investigated β-blocker therapy included longer follow-up end points to assess their efficacy. In this category, the highly publicized study in the *New England Journal of Medicine* by Mangano and colleagues was the first to suggest that perioperative β-blockade with atenolol protected against cardiac death (4% versus 12% with placebo) and all-cause mortality (9% versus 21% with placebo) for 2 years after surgery [2]. Although these results were highly promising, this study has been debated strongly because of concerns about its execution and data analysis. In another study, Poldermans and colleagues [28] followed up on an earlier bisoprolol trial in patients who had undergone vascular surgery. They demonstrated that the cardiac risk–reducing effects of bisoprolol persisted for 2 years after surgery with continued therapy (cardiac death and MI: 12% with chronic bisoprolol, 32% in controls; $P=.025$). Extending these findings, Kertai and colleagues [29] reported that long-term β-blocker use after vascular surgery was associated with an overall 70% reduction in late cardiac risk, especially in patients with a positive dobutamine stress test. Because available data are far from complete, a definitive β-blocker effect on late cardiac complications cannot be inferred, although the prospects for combined perioperative and long-term β-blockade in properly selected patients look promising. Future β-blocker trials likely will focus on deciding who, when, and how long to treat.

Clonidine

Clonidine is a selective partial agonist for α_2-adrenoreceptors that diminishes central and peripheral sympathetic outflow, in addition to activating imidazoline-preferring receptors. Intraoperative use of clonidine reduces catecholamine levels, attenuates blood pressure and heart rate responses, and reduces intraoperative myocardial ischemia. Based on previous findings that linked myocardial ischemia to increased mortality [30], Wallace and colleagues [31] conducted a prospective, double-blinded trial in 190 patients who were scheduled for noncardiac surgery to assess the role of perioperative clonidine in reducing postoperative mortality. This trial reported that a 4-day treatment protocol with clonidine reduced all-cause mortality over 2 years from 29% (placebo: 19 deaths/65 patients) to 15% (clonidine: 19 deaths/125 patients; $P=.035$; relative risk, 0.43). This clonidine effect was associated with dramatically lower postoperative serum catecholamine levels (epinephrine: 223 ± 332 pg/ml [clonidine] versus 412 ± 555 pg/ml [placebo], $P=.05$; norepinephrine: 357 ± 522 pg/ml [clonidine] versus 1054 ± 791 pg/ml [placebo], $P=.002$) and myocardial ischemia rates (day 0–3: 14% versus 31%; $P=.01$).

Statins

A recent meta-analysis of large-scale, randomized, controlled trials demonstrated that statin therapy in patients who had coronary artery disease resulted in relative risk reductions of 13% for overall mortality, 26% for fatal and nonfatal MI, and 18% for fatal and nonfatal stroke [32]. Statins lower cholesterol, but they also have important antithrombotic, anti-inflammatory, and coronary plaque-stabilizing effects [33]. These pleiotropic effects make statins ideal candidates for the treatment of chronic cardiovascular disease as well as for cardiac risk-reducing strategies in the surgical setting.

The preponderance of evidence suggests beneficial effects for statin therapy in the first 30 days after surgery, but new (albeit limited) data show that long-term survival also is improved. Kertai and colleagues [34] reported in a retrospective analysis of 510 patients who survived abdominal aortic aneurysm surgery that long-term statin users had a significantly lower prevalence of all-cause (18% versus 50%; $P<0.001$) and cardiovascular (11% versus 34%; $P<0.001$) mortality than did nonusers over a median follow-up period of 4.7 years. This effect was independent of clinical risk factors and β-blocker use. In the only prospective, randomized, placebo-controlled and double-blinded trial to date, Durazzo and colleagues [35] found that 45 days of atorvastatin therapy in patients who underwent vascular surgery (started on average 30 days before surgery) resulted in a threefold reduction (8% versus 26%; $P=.031$) in a composite of cardiovascular events (cardiac death, nonfatal MI, ischemic stroke, unstable angina) within the 6-month observation period of this study. These studies suggest that statins show considerable promise for reducing long-term complications and improving survival rates in high-risk patients who undergo vascular surgery. Further trials are awaited eagerly to confirm these findings and to evaluate combinatorial therapies of statins with other cardioprotective interventions.

Insulin therapy

Hyperglycemia at admission or in the critically ill has emerged as an independent predictor of adverse outcome [36,37]. In contrast, aggressive glucose control can reduce these complications and improve survival [38]. Acute hyperglycemia upsets a host of biologic systems, which impair critical functions of the innate immune response to infection (eg, chemotaxis, phagocytosis, production of reactive oxygen species), while enhancing certain proinflammatory processes, such as the release of proinflammatory cytokines, the expression of adhesion molecules on vascular endothelium and neutrophils, and the activation of complement [39–44]. Especially noteworthy is the interaction between advanced glycation end products (AGE), which are nonenzymatically glycosylated proteins, and their receptor (RAGE). That interaction generates potent proinflammatory signals (through nuclear factor-kappa B [NF-κB] activation), which, in turn, amplify the expression of RAGE by a positive feedback mechanism that potentially permits acute inflammation to transition into a chronic state [45,46].

In the Diabetes and Insulin Glucose Infusion in Acute Myocardial Infarction Study, Malmberg and colleagues [47] demonstrated that aggressive insulin therapy can reverse some of these negative consequences, which improves outcome in the short-term and the long-term. These investigators used a glucose–insulin infusion in diabetic patients after MI to maintain serum glucose values of less than 200 mg/dL; they demonstrated a 30% reduction in mortality that was maintained for a mean of 3.5 years. Building on these findings, Lazar and colleagues [48] studied prospectively the effects of tight glucose control on outcome in patients who underwent coronary artery bypass graft surgery, using a glucose-insulin-potassium (GIK) infusion from the time immediately before to 12 hours after surgery. Lower serum glucose values in the group that received GIK (138 ± 4 mg/dL versus 260 ± 6 mg/dL; $P < .0001$) resulted in a decreased frequency of atrial fibrillation, fewer episodes of recurrent ischemia, fewer wound infections, and improved survival in the 2 years after surgery. As intensive insulin therapy finds its place in the perioperative and critical care setting, and as we await additional trials on the long-term benefits of this therapy, it is interesting to note that insulin itself, apart from its glucose-lowering properties, exerts a spectrum of nonmetabolic effects (eg, antiapoptotic, anti-inflammatory) that is beneficial.

Anesthetic management

A recent prospective observational study proposed a link between anesthetic management and 1-year mortality after surgery [3]. When Monk and colleagues examined demographic, preoperative clinical, surgical, and intraoperative variables from adult patients who underwent noncardiac surgery, they surprisingly identified through multivariate Cox proportional hazards modeling that "cumulative deep hypnotic time," a measure of hypnotic depth (bispectral index [BIS]<45) per hour of time, was associated independently with first-year death rates (OR, 1.24/h; $P = .012$). Another study by Lennmarken [49] came to almost the same conclusions independently. Although these results are intriguing, further research is required to address some of the inherent limitations in this work.

Neither of the trials measured total anesthetic dose; therefore, the possibility cannot be excluded that adjuvant therapies (eg, β-blockers), patient characteristics, or other factors that are unrelated to increased exposure to the anesthetic agent decreased BIS values in the high-risk group.

In weighing the findings of these studies, it is necessary to recognize their shortcomings. Some of the evidence is observational, correlative, and retrospective. Even when collected prospectively, it is not always backed by other, independent investigations. The total number of data points for many of these interventions is low, the causes of death are underreported frequently, and patient risk factors and other variables in the care environment are not always characterized sufficiently. These are indications of how difficult and costly it would be to conduct informative research into long-term outcome, with its high demands on infrastructure, patient populations, data management, and budgets. With these caveats in place, however, it also should be noted that as a whole the evidence from these studies is consistent with a sizable trend that certain elements of the perioperative process can prevent or induce complications or death beyond the 30-day mark after surgery. Stated differently, these data support the concept that some of the late complications after surgery are tied to the perioperative period and are not exclusively a consequence of the natural course of illness.

The quoted studies provide one more important insight. Despite the puzzling variety of clinical and treatment variables that seem to be operative in this long-term influence, an important commonality is their shared ability to alter outcome rates by modulating different aspects of innate or adaptive immunity. Although other mechanisms could be at play, the effects of blood transfusions and their association with TRIM, the anti-inflammatory actions of statins and insulin, and the broader effects of postoperative infections and complications on maintaining a heightened state of inflammation all point to innate or adaptive immunity.

At first glance, such an explanation does not seem to account for β-blockers and clonidine. β-Blockers presumably reduce cardiac risk by reducing stress and hemodynamic responses during surgery; however, in light of recent advances in our understanding of how specific signals of the stress response can incite inflammation, and how β-blockers can intercept these effects effectively (see the article by Bierhaus and colleagues elsewhere in this issue), it is possible that β-blockers provide an indirect anti-inflammatory shield in the context of a heightened stress response. The modulating effect of β-blockers on proinflammatory cytokine production was demonstrated in patients who had dilated cardiomyopathy and in a rat model of acute MI [50,51]. Clonidine would complement this model through its known actions of suppressing catecholamine release. This raises the intriguing possibility that increased therapeutic benefits could be seen, barring any adverse hemodynamic events, following a combinatorial therapy using both classes of drugs.

In the end, the different modifiers of long-term outcome that are presented here seem to have a larger "class effect" on immunity, which reinforces the fact that immune-mediated mechanisms could contribute importantly to the occurrence of late complications. To place better these findings in the context of the immune events of the perioperative period, the following section elaborates on the innate and adaptive immune responses and highlights promising areas for future research.

Inflammation and innate immunity

Many elements of the perioperative experience influence the immune system; an incomplete list of the more dominant factors includes such widely divergent elements as the fear of surgery, tissue injury, hypothermia, many of the anesthetic drugs, blood transfusions, pain, hyperglycemia, and infections (Fig. 1). Confronted with this storm of incoming signals, the immune system rallies to kill microbes, heal tissue, and return to homeostasis. But not all of these signals cause inflammation; some of them suppress immunity, and both conditions often exist concurrently—a concept that is not immediately intuitive to many practicing anesthesiologists. The immune response to surgery and anesthesia is necessarily complex and almost always life-preserving, but also can be detrimental. A clear delineation of these different immune states (ie, proinflammation and immunosuppression) in their respective perioperative contexts is necessary to advance the discussion of long-term risk.

Acute inflammation in the operative setting is caused predominantly by the tissue injury, infection, or both. The acute inflammatory response to surgery is primarily a product of the innate immune system. Evolutionarily ancient, innate immunity shares some of its cardinal features with plants and invertebrates, and in humans uses a variety of strategies for host defense, including anatomic (eg, skin, mucous membranes) and physiologic (temperature, pH) barriers, as well as phagocytically/endocytically active cells. In this sense, innate immunity is not limited to a few specialized cell types, yet macrophages, neutrophils, natural killer cells, mast cells, basophils, and eosinophils are indispensable for its proper function. When danger lurks, innate immunity is first to respond. Its primary task is to detect, contain, and eliminate invading microbes (bacteria, fungi, viruses) quickly, and it does so by relying on macrophages and mast cells that are stationed strategically in the tissues and circulating neutrophils to signal and engage foreign genomes. Once infection is confirmed, potent mediators are released—eicosanoids, tryptases, cytokines, proteases, chemokines, and other "go signals" of the host defense—to induce local inflammation, coagulation, and controlled tissue destruction in the interest of preventing microbial spread and survival. Without infection, aseptic tissue injury unfolds a similar pattern of innate immune reactions, in part because broken cells release compounds like heat shock proteins, mitochondrial proteins, and the transcription factor high mobility group 1 (HMGB1) into the extracellular environment. The fight against microbes and the natural closure of a wound depend critically on a carefully regulated innate immune system [52].

When locally controlled host defenses become systemic, a heightened inflammatory response can cause organ damage or death, a fact that is well appreciated

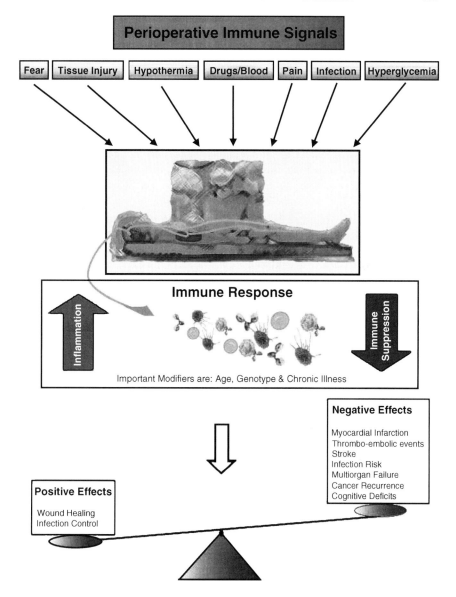

Fig. 1. The perioperative immune response. The immune system responds to multiple signals from the perioperative period to preserve life, heal tissue, and fight infection. When the immune response becomes unbalanced in the course of major surgery, trauma, or sepsis, heightened inflammation and suppressed immunity can cause acute autotoxicity, delayed complications, or death.

in patients who suffer from trauma, burn injury, and sepsis. Although less extreme, systemic inflammation also can be induced by major surgery, with its severity proportional to the degree of tissue injury and the length of surgery [53,54]. Soluble factors of the inflammatory response recruit other systems into the mix, which activate coagulation and the stress response; in turn, these generate signals to escalate the underlying inflammatory state [55,56]. It should come as no surprise that—in the context of long-term risk—a systemic condition that is marked by high catecholamines, inflammation, and procoagulation could fuel the progression of certain chronic inflammatory diseases, and that the severity (amplitude and duration) of this inflammatory response, as well as the stage (or activity) of the underlying chronic illness, are important variables in this interaction.

The concept of disease activity is critical as illustrated by recent insights that coronary plaque vulnerability, or the inflammatory activity of the plaque, is a more important determinant of plaque rupture than the size of the lesion alone, which could be large, but well encased by a stable fibrotic cap [57,58]. Therefore, therapeutic efforts can be divided conceptually into those that seek to control the host response (eg, perioperative opioids, β-blockers, clonidine) and those that attempt to stabilize disease activity preoperatively (eg, statin use or glucose control days and weeks before surgery). Even in well-studied areas like postoperative MI, we lack a basic understanding at the cellular and molecular level of the factors that promote the acute destabilization of the coronary plaque and perioperative plaque rupture. Little is known as well about how the acute host response to surgery affects the symptomatology and progression of many other chronic inflammatory or autoimmune diseases. These areas are ripe for scientific inquiry. The paucity of data is due, in part, to the lack of suitable animal models, but can be explained additionally by the vast complexity of multiple interacting biologic pathways, which makes identifying culprit events (or specific cell signals) a daunting task. Several new studies, however, indicate that significant progress is being made.

Interleukin-6 and C-reactive protein

Among the many "surgical cytokines" that have been measured in the context of major surgery and trauma, the pleiotropic interleukin (IL)-6 and the acute-phase reactant C-reactive protein (CRP) are elevated most consistently in the perioperative setting [59–61]. Referred to as "markers of the inflammatory response," these two entities have potent and essential biologic activities. IL-6 increases quickly within a few hours of surgery, peaks during the first two postoperative days, and acting as a hepatocyte-stimulating factor, induces the synthesis of CRP, fibrinogen, and other acute-phase reactants [62]. IL-6 is a pleiotropic cytokine with proinflammatory, anti-inflammatory, and immune-modulatory activities that plays an important role in the progression of coronary artery disease [63,64]. Overproduction of IL-6 is involved in the pathology of several chronic inflammatory diseases, such as rheumatoid arthritis, Crohn's disease, and juvenile idiopathic arthritis [65]. Furthermore, IL-6 is—by all indications—the principal cytokine that is responsible for tissue factor–dependent thrombin generation, and therefore, acts as a key link in the bidirectional relation between inflammation and coagulation [66].

The Perioperative Genetics and Safety Outcomes Study Investigative Team at Duke is reporting that patients with coincident polymorphisms in two minor alleles of the IL-6 (-174G/C) and CRP (3'UTR 1846C/T) genes experience a threefold increase in stroke risk after cardiac surgery [67]. Functionally, these common gene variants result in higher expression levels of their respective proteins and previously were associated with other perioperative inflammatory complications [68,69]. Individual genetic profiles, as assessed by polymorphisms, and their link to inflammation risk also should provide important insights into the biology of long-term outcome.

Until more detailed "maps" of these interacting factors are assembled, and new therapies emerge, our best chance at minimizing acute inflammatory response is to improve surgical technique (eg, minimally invasive surgery) to reduce tissue injury and to manage anesthesia carefully by assessing and preparing the patient in the preoperative period and implementing evidence-based risk-reducing drug therapies; controlling the intraoperative stress response and preventing excessive physiologic and metabolic "swings"; meticulously controlling infection; and managing pain postoperatively. These efforts not only define the modern standard of anesthesia care, but also seem to be especially relevant in light of the aforementioned association between early postoperative complications and long-term mortality.

Immunosuppression and adaptive immunity

A didactic separation of the innate and adaptive immunity has its role today, as indeed it has had in the history of immunology research, with Ilya Metchnikoff's phagocytosis theory and Paul Ehrlich's theory on the specificity of immunity; both won the Nobel Prize in Physiology and Medicine in 1908. We must recognize that the two systems are highly integrated and instruct and regulate each other in the constant struggle to discriminate self from nonself. These reciprocal links between innate and adaptive immunity have important functional consequences in determining the amplitude and resolution of the inflammatory response and the state of immunosuppression after major surgery and injury. Only fairly recently has research in the context of surgery and trauma begun to place itself at this interface of the immune system, but the results have been promising and indicate that much more work is needed here [70].

Around 450 million years ago, a germline insertion of predecessors of the recombinase-activating genes RAG-1 and RAG-2 made possible the evolution of the adaptive immune system, which makes it phylogenetically much younger than innate immunity [71]. What evolved is a highly complex system of two major populations of lymphocytes—B lymphocytes (B cells) and T lymphocytes (T cells)—that can bind to small regions (epitopes) of microbial molecules (antigenic specificity), recognize them as foreign (self/nonself recognition), and remember their "barcode" for future encounters (immunologic memory). But evolution did not dismiss the older, innate immune system, and instead endowed it with critical roles in the presentation of antigen and the expression of costimulatory signals to guide the primary adaptive immune response [72].

Many of these functions are altered by major surgery, and it seems that anesthetic management takes an active role in this process. Following the initial spike of inflammatory activity that is due to major surgery or trauma, a secondary stage of suppressed immune activity comes into play, in part to counteract the effects of the initial host response. In this secondary phase, monocytes are tolerant to endotoxin and do not secrete normal amounts of proinflammatory cytokines [73,74], antigen presentation is suppressed, natural killer cell function is compromised (eg, decreased interferon-γ production) [75], the total number of blood lymphocytes is decreased [76], and the so-called "T helper lymphocyte 1 to T helper lymphocyte 2 (Th1/Th2) balance" is lopsided toward the anti-inflammatory/immunosuppressive Th2 cytokine profile (IL-4, IL-5, IL-6, IL-10, IL-13) [77].

Several studies in the anesthesia literature indicate that volatile anesthetics may contribute to these conditions. Clinically relevant doses of several volatile anesthetics suppressed inducible nitric oxide synthase expression and nitric oxide production in macrophages. Other studies showed that natural killer cell cytotoxicity is depressed in mice that are exposed to halothane and isoflurane. Inhalational anesthetics also seem to induce programmed cell death in lymphocytes, depress lymphocyte function, and alter the distribution of lymphocyte subsets [78–81]. Anesthesia and surgery have a compounding "immune paralytic" effect, which puts patients at risk for nosocomial infections and possibly for tumor recurrence through impaired immune surveillance.

Intrinsic modifiers of the immune response

In the foregoing discussion, predominant consideration was given to the external elements that engage the immune system during surgery and anesthesia, whereas less attention was paid to intrinsic host factors. If we presume that the kinetics of the inflammatory response (height, duration) have a determining influence on long-term risk, intrinsic host factors become critical in an immune system that is highly vulnerable to interference because it relies on a complex set of rules to maintain a state of high alert, as well as on active countermeasures to prevent false starts and toxic overreactivity. It is becoming increasingly clear that host genetic diversity, often modified by environmental conditions, exerts a strong influence on the tonic state and responsiveness of the immune system. A series of well over 50 gene mutations has been described to result in spontaneous, chronic inflammation in otherwise unchallenged mice (Table 1).

It is only reasonable to assume that many more genetic determinants of the host response will be identified, which will have important clinical relevance in regulating the immune output to infection and injury. The recently discovered association between a tumor necrosis factor α gene polymorphism, enhanced inflammatory response, and worsened outcome after cardiopulmonary bypass [82], and the aforementioned report on IL-6 and CRP genetic variants by the Duke University group [67] are cogent examples of what lies ahead. Although in our specialty we may find it more intuitive to study inherited variations in genes that predict drug response, we also must pay careful attention to, and contribute, to the field of immunogenomics because it likely will yield equally dramatic results.

The genetic predisposition to microbial pathogens will be relevant to infectious disease susceptibility, severity, and outcome in the perioperative period and the surgical ICUs. Well-known examples of this genetic influence in the nonsurgical setting include the enhanced resistance to malaria in heterozygous carriers of the sickle gene mutation [83], and the protection against HIV infection in individuals homozygous for a deletion mutation in the chemokine receptor CCR5 [84]; however, evidence is accumulating rapidly that polymorphisms in genes that encode human leukocyte antigens, complement components, Toll-like receptors, mannose-binding lectin, and others are affecting host susceptibility to acute bacterial infections. In one such example, Kotb and colleagues [85] from the University of Tennessee identified different HLA class II haplotypes that protect against or predispose to invasive Group A streptococcal infections.

Beyond genetics, there is now evidence from the author's laboratory and the work of James Lederer and his group at the Brigham that nongenetic acquisition of harmful, dysregulated immune responses to microbial constituents can evolve in the context of acute injury or chronic illness. These effects seem to be mediated through the Toll-like receptor (TLR) system. In a seminal 1989 article, Charles Janeway, Jr. predicted that the innate immune system uses what he called "pattern recognition receptors" to detect infection through the recognition of evolutionarily conserved microbial constituents, also called pathogen-associated molecular patterns (PAMPs), which are invariant among pathogens of a given class, and thus, are the basis for self–nonself discrimination [86]. His vision was confirmed in 1997 through the discovery of the first mammalian homolog of the *Drosophila* Toll protein (TLR), which had been known to be involved critically in the fly's defense against fungal infections [87]. Since then, the human family of TLRs has grown to 11 members, and is capable of sensing a wide spectrum of microbial ligands (eg, lipopolysaccharide [LPS], peptidoglycan, flagellin, and many others). Beyond the ability to sense PAMPs, TLRs orchestrate an offensive inflammatory response through the activation of the signal transducer NF-κB and Mitogen-activated protein kinase signaling, as well as being critically involved in initiating the subsequent wave of adaptive immune responses. Intriguingly, evidence now exists that TLRs also can recognize endogenous ligands that are induced during the inflammatory response (eg, heat shock proteins, hyaluronic acid, fibronectin), a setting in which certain TLRs may evoke an exaggerated

270 MEILER

Table 1
Products encoded by genes whose disruption or mutation leads to spontaneous inflammation

Gene products	Human (H) Mouse (M)	Inflammatory phenotype	Predominant sites
Factors directly involved in regulation of apoptosis			
Fas (CD95)	H	Urticarial rash, glomerulonephritis, oral ulceration, lymphocyte infiltration	Skin, kidney, mouth, liver
Fas (CD95) (lpr)	M	Glomerulonephritis, necrotizing vasculitis, erosive synovitis, interstitial pneumonitis, dermatitis	Kidney, mesentery, joints, lung, skin, vessels
Factors believed to be involved in clearance of immune complexes and material from apoptotic cells			
C1q (A, B and C genes)	H	Rash, glomerulonephritis, oral ulceration	Skin, kidney, mouth
C1q (a gene)	M	Glomerulonephritis	Kidney
C2	H	Rash, vasculitis, arthritis, glomerulonephritis, asthma	Skin, joints, lung
C4	H	Rash	Skin
C4	M	Glomerulonephritis	Kidney
C3	H	Glomerulonephritis	Kidney
C4-binding protein	H	Ulcerations	Mouth
Factor H	H	Glomerulonephritis, rash	Kidney, skin
Crry	M	Neutrophil infiltration	Placenta
Serum amyloid P component	M	Glomerulonephritis	Kidney
DNase I	M	Glomerulonephritis	Kidney
FcγRIIB	M	Glomerulonephritis	Kidney
WASP (Wiskott-Aldrich syndrome protein)	H	Eczema, vasculitis, renal disease, arthritis, inflammatory bowel disease	Skin, kidney, joints, bowels
Cytokines, cytokine receptors, and other cell surface receptors			
WASP	M	Lymphocyte and neutrophil infiltration	Colon
TNF-R1 (tumor-necrosis factor receptor 1)	H	Familial Hibernian fever (periodic fever, conjunctivitis, periorbital edema, arthralgia)	Systemic, eyes, joints

TGF-β1 (transforming growth factor-β1)	M	Macrophage, lymphocyte and neutrophil infiltration in blood vessels and parenchyma; gastric ulceration	Lung, heart, stomach, liver spleen, lymph nodes, pancreas, colon, salivary glands, striated muscle
IL-2Rα (interleukin-2 receptor-α)	M	Lymphocyte and neutrophil infiltration; ulceration	Colon
IL-2	M	Granulocyte, lymphocyte and plasma cell infiltration; ulceration	Colon
IL-10	M	Lymphocyte and neutrophil infiltration	Duodenum, jejunum, ileum, colon
GM-CSF (granulocyte-macrophage colony-stimulating factor)	M	Lymphocyte infiltration around airways and veins	Lung
IL-1Ra (IL-1 receptor antagonist)	M	Neutrophil, macrophage and CD4$^+$ lymphocyte infiltration	Aorta, coronaries, iliac and popliteal arteries
IL-1Ra	M	Erosive arthritis	Joints
T-cell receptor-α	M	γδ T-cell, B-cell, plasma cell and neutrophil infiltration	Colon
T-cell receptor-β	M	γδ T-cell, B-cell, plasma cell and neutrophil infiltration	Colon
Major histocompatibility complex class II	M	Lymphocyte and neutrophil infiltration	Colon
CTLA4 (cytotoxic T-lymphocyte antigen 4)	M	Lymphocyte, macrophage, and granulocyte infiltration	Heart, pancreas, lung, bone marrow, liver, salivary glands, joints, blood vessels
PD-1	M	Arthritis, glomerulonephritis, carditis	Joints, kidneys, heart
Intracellular factor in lymphocytes, leukocytes, and epithelial cells affecting their activation			
LAT (linker for activation of T cells)	M	CD4$^+$ T-cell, eosinophil, B-cell and macrophage infiltration	Multiple organs
SOCS1 (suppressor of cytokine signaling)	M	Macrophage infiltration	Liver, lungs, pancreas, heart, skin
Phosphatidylinositol 3-phosphate kinase p110δ	M	Leukocyte infiltration	Cecum, rectum
Pten (Phosphatase active on PtdIns(3,4,5)P$_3$)	M	Inflammatory interstitial infiltration	Lung
Lyn	M	Glomerulonephritis, renal capillary vasculitis	Kidney

(continued on next page)

Table 1 (*continued*)

Gene products	Human (H) Mouse (M)	Inflammatory phenotype	Predominant sites
Intracellular factor in lymphocytes, leukocytes, and epithelial cells affecting their activation			
Cbl	M	Activated B- and T-cell infiltration	Salivary glands, pancreas, liver, intestine, lung, kidney, heart, skeletal muscle, urinary bladder
$G\alpha_{i2}$	M	Lymphocyte, plasma cell and neutrophil infiltration; ulceration	Colon
SHP-1 (protein tyrosine phosphatase)	M	Neutrophil abscesses, interstitial pneumonitis	Skin, lung
SHIP (inositol-5-phosphatase)	M	Macrophage infiltration	Lungs
p21	M	Leukocyte infiltration, glomerulonephritis	Kidney
Tristetraproline	M	Neutrophil, macrophage and lymphocyte infiltration; pannus formation; bone erosion; glomerulonephritis	Skin, conjunctivae, joints, kidney
NFAT (nuclear factor of activated T cells) – p and NFAT4 (double deletion)	M	Lymphocyte, macrophage, plasma cell, neutrophil, and mast cell infiltration	Eyelids, lungs
IKK (IĸB kinase)-2 (deficiency restricted to keratinocytes)	M	Macrophage, neutrophil and CD4$^+$ T-cell infiltration	Skin
IKKγ (NEMO: NF-kB essential modulator)	H	Rash; eosinophil and neutrophil infiltration	Skin
IKKγ (NEMO: NF-kB essential modulator)	M	Neutrophil and eosinophil infiltration; iNOS expression	Skin
I kBα (inhibitor of NF- kB)	M	Neutrophil abscesses and macrophage infiltration	Skin
E 3 ubiquitin ligase	M	Macrophage and plasma cell infiltration; fibrosis; alveolar proteinosis	Lung
RelB	M	T-cell, eosinophil, neutrophil, macrophage and mast cell infiltration; collagen deposition; hyperplasia of mucus-secreting cells	Skin, lungs, liver, salivary glands, skeletal muscles, stomach, epididymis, ovaries, uterus
NF-kB1 (p105)(retaining p50)	M	Lymphocyte infiltration around vessels, portal tracts and airways	Lungs, liver

T-bet	M	Peribronchial and perivenular eosinophil and lymphocyte infiltration; collagen deposition	Lungs
Gadd45a (growth arrest and DNA damage-inducible gene)	M	Glomerulonephritis, perivascular mononuclear infiltration	Kidney
Mdr (multiple drug resistance)-1a	M	CD4+ T-cell, B-cell and granulocyte infiltration; mucosal thickening and ulceration	Colon
NOD2/CARD15	H	Crohn's disease (granulomas, fibrosis)	Ileum
NOD2/CARD15	H	Blau syndrome (granulomatous arthritis, uveitis, rash)	Joints, eyes, skin
Pyrin	H	Familial Mediterranean fever (fever, neutrophil infiltration)	Systemic, joints, peritoneum, pleural space
Cryopyrin or CIAS (cold-induced autoinflammatory syndrome)-1	H	Cold-induced periodic fever, rash, arthralgia, conjunctivitis; or without cold induction (Muckle-Wells syndrome)	Systemic, skin, joints, conjunctivae
Mevalonate kinase	H	Periodic fever, arthralgia, abdominal pain, rash	Systemic, joints, peritoneum (?), skin
Factors affecting oxidative stress			
Haem oxygenase 1	M	Lymphocyte, neutrophil and macrophage infiltration;fibrosis; glomerulonephritis	Liver, lung, kidney
Surfactant protein D	M	Monocyte peribronchiolar and perivascular infiltration; emphysema	Lung

Spontaneous indicates substantially more frequent occurrence than in wild-type hosts, despite lack of known infection or experimental intervention, in subjects living under normal conditions, presumably with normal gastrointestinal flora. People who have Wiskott-Aldrich syndrome experience frequent infections but the disorder is included for comparison with the mutant mouse, in which infections have not been described. Only inflammatory aspects of the phenotype are listed, even when these are not the major manifestations of the disorder. Abnormal accumulation of lymphocytes in lymphoid organs and the development of autoantibodies are not considered signs of inflammation. Entries are omitted for disorders in which the mutated gene has not been identified; the mutation is believed to confer a gain of function; the phenotype requires that two known genes be mutated; or only a single case has been reported. For mice, the phenotype is described in the strain background in which it is most pronounced, provided that the background does not furnish another known mutation with a related phenotype.

Modified from Nathan C. Points of inflammation. Nature 2002;420(6917):846–52.

(and harmful) release of proinflammatory mediators in response to an acute, superimposed infection. In an elegant series of studies, Lederer's group reported that thermal injury in mice was associated with an exaggerated response to LPSs, which caused profound hypercytokinemia and high mortality compared with control animals. This response required several days to develop and in all likelihood was mediated by enhanced TLR4 (part of the LPS receptor complex) reactivity [88–90]. The author's findings parallel these observations on an even more dramatic scale, using sickle cell disease in mice as a model of a chronic inflammatory disease (unpublished data). Taken together, these results suggest that—independent of genetic influence—immune dysregulation can evolve in the setting of acute injury or certain chronic inflammatory conditions, and is sufficient to amplify the response to acute, superimposed infectious signals with potentially devastating consequences to the host.

Summary

There is a strong possibility that the risk from anesthesia and surgery carries over from the immediate perioperative period to more remote time points. This extended risk seems to influence the progression, severity, and complication rate of certain chronic illnesses, such as vascular heart disease and some of the malignancies, although other disease processes might be affected as well. With the recognition that the perioperative process could be responsible for later adverse events comes the need to reassess existing patient safety models, because some of the risk could be preventable. To confront these challenges, it is necessary to understand the underlying biology of this association, and immunology should be particularly helpful in this pursuit. It will be of special importance to integrate our knowledge of the host immune response to anesthesia and surgery with the recent revelations on the role of immunity in the progression of many of the chronic diseases. Additionally, we need to examine how genetic diversity or acquired defects alter the immune response to tissue injury and infection so that we can improve risk stratification and preemptive therapies. In the meantime, we must strive to improve short- and long-term outcomes by expanding our efforts to reduce disease activity preoperatively, to control the surgical stress response and infection rate, and to use tissue-preserving surgical techniques. Long-term patient safety after anesthesia and surgery is not a specialty-by-specialty endeavor; it requires a highly collaborative, institutional, and national effort to foster innovative research and health care process improvements.

Acknowledgments

The author thanks Kimberly McGhee and Kavitha Krishnarao for assistance in preparing this manuscript.

References

[1] Gaba DM. Meeting report: anesthesia, surgery, and long-term outcomes. September 21–22, 2004. Available at: http://www.apsf.org/assets/Documents/APSF_LTO_Wkshop_Report.pdf. Accessed March 5, 2006.

[2] Mangano DT, Layug EL, Wallace A, et al. Effect of atenolol on mortality and cardiovascular morbidity after noncardiac surgery. Multicenter Study of Perioperative Ischemia Research Group. N Engl J Med 1996;335(23):1713–20.

[3] Monk TG, Saini V, Weldon BC, et al. Anesthetic management and one-year mortality after noncardiac surgery. Anesth Analg 2005;100(1):4–10.

[4] Aharonoff GB, Koval KJ, Skovron ML, et al. Hip fractures in the elderly: predictors of one year mortality. J Orthop Trauma 1997;11(3):162–5.

[5] Lagasse RS. Anesthesia safety: model or myth? A review of the published literature and analysis of current original data. Anesthesiology 2002;97(6):1609–17.

[6] Khuri SF, Daley J, Henderson W, et al. Risk adjustment of the postoperative mortality rate for the comparative assessment of the quality of surgical care: results of the National Veterans Affairs Surgical Risk Study. J Am Coll Surg 1997;185(4):315–27.

[7] Meiler SE. Can we alter long-term outcome? The role of anesthetic management and the inflammatory response. Anesthesia Patient Safety Foundation Newsletter 2003;18(3):33,35.

[8] Meiler SE. Can we alter long-term outcome? The role of inflammation and immunity in the perioperative period (Part II). Anesthesia Patient Safety Foundation Newsletter 2004;19(1): 1,3–4,7.

[9] Casserly I, Topol E. Convergence of atherosclerosis and Alzheimer's disease: inflammation, cholesterol, and misfolded proteins. Lancet 2004;363(9415):1139–46.

[10] Salo M. Effects of anesthesia and surgery on the immune response. Acta Anaesthesiol Scand 1992;36(3):201–20.

[11] Committee on Quality of Health Care in America IOM. In: Kohn L, Corrigan J, Donaldson M, editors. To err is human: building a safer health system. Washington DC: National Academy Press; 1999.

[12] Opelz G, Sengar DP, Mickey MR, et al. Effect of blood transfusions on subsequent kidney transplants. Transplant Proc 1973;5(1):253–9.

[13] Opelz G, Terasaki PI. Improvement of kidney-graft survival with increased numbers of blood transfusions. N Engl J Med 1978;299(15):799–803.

[14] Sanfilippo F, Spees EK, Vaughn WK. The timing of pretransplant transfusions and renal allograft survival. Transplantation 1984;37(4):344–50.

[15] Opelz G, Vanrenterghem Y, Kirste G, et al. Prospective evaluation of pretransplant blood transfusions in cadaver kidney recipients. Transplantation 1997;63(7):964–7.

[16] Fischer E, Lenhard V, Seifert P, et al. Blood transfusion-induced suppression of cellular immunity in man. Hum Immunol 1980;1(3):187–94.

[17] Quigley RL, Wood KJ, Morris PJ. Transfusion induces blood donor-specific suppressor cells. J Immunol 1989;142(2):463–70.

[18] de Waal LP, van Twuyver E. Blood transfusion and allograft survival: is mixed chimerism the solution for tolerance induction in clinical transplantation? Crit Rev Immunol 1991;10(5): 417–25.

[19] Terasaki PI. The beneficial transfusion effect on kidney graft survival attributed to clonal deletion. Transplantation 1984;37(2):119–25.

[20] Opelz G, Mickey MR, Terasaki PI. Identification of unresponsive kidney-transplant recipients. Lancet 1972;1(7756):868–71.

[21] Blajchman MA. Immunomodulation and blood transfusion. Am J Ther 2002;9(5):389–95.

[22] Brand A. Immunological aspects of blood transfusions. Transpl Immunol 2002;10(2–3):183–90.

[23] Hill GE, Frawley WH, Griffith KE, et al. Allogeneic blood transfusion increases the risk of postoperative bacterial infection: a meta-analysis. J Trauma 2003;54(5):908–14.

[24] Amato A, Pescatori M. Perioperative blood transfusions for the recurrence of colorectal cancer [review]. Cochrane Database Syst Rev 2006;(1):CD005033.

[25] Vamvakas EC. White-blood-cell-containing allogeneic blood transfusion, postoperative infection and mortality: a meta-analysis of observational 'before-and-after' studies. Vox Sang 2004;86(2): 111–9.

[26] Thurer RL, Luban NL, AuBuchon JP, et al. Universal WBC reduction. Transfusion 2000;40(6): 751–2.

[27] Khuri SF, Henderson WG, DePalma RG, et al. Determinants of long-term survival after major surgery and the adverse effect of postoperative complications. Ann Surg 2005;242(3):326–41 [discussion 341-3].

[28] Poldermans D, Boersma E, Bax JJ, et al. Bisoprolol reduces cardiac death and myocardial infarction in high-risk patients as long as 2 years after successful major vascular surgery. Eur Heart J 2001;22(15):1353–8.

[29] Kertai MD, Boersma E, Bax JJ, et al. Optimizing long-term cardiac management after major vascular surgery: Role of beta-blocker therapy, clinical characteristics, and dobutamine stress echocardiography to optimize long-term cardiac management after major vascular surgery. Arch Intern Med 2003;163(18):2230–5.

[30] Wallace A, Layug B, Tateo I, et al. Prophylactic atenolol reduces postoperative myocardial ischemia. McSPI Research Group. Anesthesiology 1998;88(1):7–17.

[31] Wallace AW, Galindez D, Salahieh A, et al. Effect of clonidine on cardiovascular morbidity and mortality after noncardiac surgery. Anesthesiology 2004;101(2):284–93.

[32] Briel M, Nordmann AJ, Bucher HC. Statin therapy for prevention and treatment of acute and chronic cardiovascular disease: update on recent trials and metaanalyses. Curr Opin Lipidol 2005;16(6):601–5.

[33] Jain MK, Ridker PM. Anti-inflammatory effects of statins: clinical evidence and basic mechanisms. Nat Rev Drug Discov 2005;4(12):977–87.

[34] Kertai MD, Boersma E, Westerhout CM, et al. Association between long-term statin use and mortality after successful abdominal aortic aneurysm surgery. Am J Med 2004;116(2):96–103.

[35] Durazzo AE, Machado FS, Ikeoka DT, et al. Reduction in cardiovascular events after vascular surgery with atorvastatin: a randomized trial. J Vasc Surg 2004;39(5):967–75 [discussion 975-6].

[36] Finney SJ, Zekveld C, Elia A, et al. Glucose control and mortality in critically ill patients. JAMA 2003;290(15):2041–7.

[37] Umpierrez GE, Isaacs SD, Bazargan N, et al. Hyperglycemia: an independent marker of in-hospital mortality in patients with undiagnosed diabetes. J Clin Endocrinol Metab 2002; 87(3):978–82.

[38] van den Berghe G, Wouters P, Weekers F, et al. Intensive insulin therapy in the critically ill patients. N Engl J Med 2001;345(19):1359–67.

[39] Marhoffer W, Stein M, Maeser E, et al. Impairment of polymorphonuclear leukocyte function and metabolic control of diabetes. Diabetes Care 1992;15(2):256–60.

[40] Wierusz-Wysocka B, Wysocki H, Wykretowicz A, et al. The influence of increasing glucose concentrations on selected functions of polymorphonuclear neutrophils. Acta Diabetol Lat 1988;25(4):283–8.

[41] Alexiewicz JM, Kumar D, Smogorzewski M, et al. Polymorphonuclear leukocytes in non-insulin-dependent diabetes mellitus: abnormalities in metabolism and function. Ann Intern Med 1995;123(12):919–24.

[42] Nielson CP, Hindson DA. Inhibition of polymorphonuclear leukocyte respiratory burst by elevated glucose concentrations in vitro. Diabetes 1989;38(8):1031–5.

[43] Dhindsa S, Tripathy D, Mohanty P, et al. Differential effects of glucose and alcohol on reactive oxygen species generation and intranuclear nuclear factor-kappaB in mononuclear cells. Metabolism 2004;53(3):330–4.

[44] Esposito K, Nappo F, Marfella R, et al. Inflammatory cytokine concentrations are acutely increased by hyperglycemia in humans: role of oxidative stress. Circulation 2002;106(16): 2067–72.

[45] Hofmann MA, Drury S, Fu C, et al. RAGE mediates a novel proinflammatory axis: a central cell surface receptor for S100/calgranulin polypeptides. Cell 1999;97(7):889–901.

[46] Yan SF, Ramasamy R, Naka Y, et al. Glycation, inflammation, and RAGE: a scaffold for the macrovascular complications of diabetes and beyond. Circ Res 2003;93(12):1159–69.

[47] Malmberg K, Norhammar A, Wedel H, et al. Glycometabolic state at admission: important risk marker of mortality in conventionally treated patients with diabetes mellitus and acute myocardial infarction: long-term results from the Diabetes and Insulin-Glucose Infusion in Acute Myocardial Infarction (DIGAMI) study. Circulation 1999;99(20):2626–32.

[48] Lazar HL, Chipkin SR, Fitzgerald CA, et al. Tight glycemic control in diabetic coronary artery bypass graft patients improves perioperative outcomes and decreases recurrent ischemic events. Circulation 2004;109(12):1497–502.

[49] Lennmarken C. Confirmation that low intraoperative BIS levels predict increased risk of postoperative mortality. Anesthesiology 2003;99:A303.

[50] Deten A, Volz HC, Holzl A, et al. Effect of propranolol on cardiac cytokine expression after myocardial infarction in rats. Mol Cell Biochem 2003;251(1–2):127–37.

[51] Ohtsuka T, Hamada M, Hiasa G, et al. Effect of beta-blockers on circulating levels of inflammatory and anti-inflammatory cytokines in patients with dilated cardiomyopathy. J Am Coll Cardiol 2001;37(2):412–7.

[52] Nathan C. Points of control in inflammation. Nature 2002;420(6917):846–52.

[53] Shenkin A, Fraser WD, Series J, et al. The serum interleukin 6 response to elective surgery. Lymphokine Res 1989;8(2):123–7.

[54] Cruickshank AM, Fraser WD, Burns HJ, et al. Response of serum interleukin-6 in patients undergoing elective surgery of varying severity. Clin Sci (Lond) 1990;79(2):161–5.

[55] Levi M, van der Poll T, Buller HR. Bidirectional relation between inflammation and coagulation. Circulation 2004;109(22):2698–704.

[56] Bokarewa MI, Morrissey JH, Tarkowski A. Tissue factor as a proinflammatory agent. Arthritis Res 2002;4(3):190–5.

[57] Libby P. Act local, act global: inflammation and the multiplicity of "vulnerable" coronary plaques. J Am Coll Cardiol 2005;45(10):1600–2.

[58] Libby P. Inflammation in atherosclerosis. Nature 2002;420(6917):868–74.

[59] Parry-Billings M, Baigrie RJ, Lamont PM, et al. Effects of major and minor surgery on plasma glutamine and cytokine levels. Arch Surg 1992;127(10):1237–40.

[60] Baigrie RJ, Lamont PM, Kwiatkowski D, et al. Systemic cytokine response after major surgery. Br J Surg 1992;79(8):757–60.

[61] Desborough JP. The stress response to trauma and surgery. Br J Anaesth 2000;85(1):109–17.

[62] Gauldie J, Richards C, Harnish D, et al. Interferon beta 2/B-cell stimulatory factor type 2 shares identity with monocyte-derived hepatocyte-stimulating factor and regulates the major acute phase protein response in liver cells. Proc Natl Acad Sci U S A 1987;84(20):7251–5.

[63] Yudkin JS, Kumari M, Humphries SE, et al. Inflammation, obesity, stress and coronary heart disease: is interleukin-6 the link? Atherosclerosis 2000;148(2):209–14.

[64] Kanda T, Takahashi T. Interleukin-6 and cardiovascular diseases. Jpn Heart J 2004;45(2):183–93.

[65] Nishimoto N, Kishimoto T, Yoshizaki K. Anti-interleukin 6 receptor antibody treatment in rheumatic disease. Ann Rheum Dis 2000;59(Suppl 1):i21–7.

[66] Levi M, van der Poll T, ten Cate H, et al. The cytokine-mediated imbalance between coagulant and anticoagulant mechanisms in sepsis and endotoxaemia. Eur J Clin Invest 1997;27(1):3–9.

[67] Grocott HP, White WD, Morris RW, et al. Genetic polymorphisms and the risk of stroke after cardiac surgery. Stroke 2005;36(9):1854–8.

[68] Gaudino M, Di Castelnuovo A, Zamparelli R, et al. Genetic control of postoperative systemic inflammatory reaction and pulmonary and renal complications after coronary artery surgery. J Thorac Cardiovasc Surg 2003;126(4):1107–12.

[69] Burzotta F, Iacoviello L, Di Castelnuovo A, et al. Relation of the -174 G/C polymorphism of interleukin-6 to interleukin-6 plasma levels and to length of hospitalization after surgical coronary revascularization. Am J Cardiol 2001;88(10):1125–8.

[70] Murphy TJ, Choileain NN, Zang Y, et al. CD4+CD25+ regulatory T cells control innate immune reactivity after injury. J Immunol 2005;174(5):2957–63.

[71] Agrawal A, Eastman QM, Schatz DG. Transposition mediated by RAG1 and RAG2 and its implications for the evolution of the immune system. Nature 1998;394(6695):744–51.
[72] Hoebe K, Janssen E, Beutler B. The interface between innate and adaptive immunity. Nat Immunol 2004;5(10):971–4.
[73] Docke WD, Randow F, Syrbe U, et al. Monocyte deactivation in septic patients: restoration by IFN-gamma treatment. Nat Med 1997;3(6):678–81.
[74] Faist E, Schinkel C, Zimmer S. Update on the mechanisms of immune suppression of injury and immune modulation. World J Surg 1996;20(4):454–9.
[75] Yadavalli GK, Auletta JJ, Gould MP, et al. Deactivation of the innate cellular immune response following endotoxic and surgical injury. Exp Mol Pathol 2001;71(3):209–21.
[76] Dietz A, Heimlich F, Daniel V, et al. Immunomodulating effects of surgical intervention in tumors of the head and neck. Otolaryngol Head Neck Surg 2000;123(1 Pt 1):132–9.
[77] Hensler T, Hecker H, Heeg K, et al. Distinct mechanisms of immunosuppression as a consequence of major surgery. Infect Immun 1997;65(6):2283–91.
[78] Matsuoka H, Kurosawa S, Horinouchi T, et al. Inhalation anesthetics induce apoptosis in normal peripheral lymphocytes in vitro. Anesthesiology 2001;95(6):1467–72.
[79] Karabiyik L, Sardas S, Polat U, et al. Comparison of genotoxicity of sevoflurane and isoflurane in human lymphocytes studied in vivo using the comet assay. Mutat Res 2001;492(1–2):99–107.
[80] Brand JM, Kirchner H, Poppe C, et al. The effects of general anesthesia on human peripheral immune cell distribution and cytokine production. Clin Immunol Immunopathol 1997;83(2):190–4.
[81] Corsi M, Mariconti P, Calvillo L, et al. Influence of inhalational, neuroleptic and local anesthesia on lymphocyte subset distribution. Int J Tissue React 1995;17(5–6):211–7.
[82] Tomasdottir H, Hjartarson H, Ricksten A, et al. Tumor necrosis factor gene polymorphism is associated with enhanced systemic inflammatory response and increased cardiopulmonary morbidity after cardiac surgery. Anesth Analg 2003;97(4):944–9.
[83] Weatherall DJ, Bell JI, Clegg JB, et al. Genetic factors as determinants of infectious disease transmission in human communities. Philos Trans R Soc Lond B Biol Sci 1988;321(1207):327–48.
[84] McNicholl JM, Smith DK, Qari SH, et al. Host genes and HIV: the role of the chemokine receptor gene CCR5 and its allele. Emerg Infect Dis 1997;3(3):261–71.
[85] Kotb M, Norrby-Teglund A, McGeer A, et al. Association of human leukocyte antigen with outcomes of infectious diseases: the streptococcal experience. Scand J Infect Dis 2003;35(9):665–9.
[86] Janeway Jr CA. Approaching the asymptote? Evolution and revolution in immunology. Cold Spring Harb Symp Quant Biol 1989;54(Pt 1):1–13.
[87] Medzhitov R, Preston-Hurlburt P, Janeway Jr CA. A human homolog of the *Drosophila* Toll protein signals activation of adaptive immunity. Nature 1997;388(6640):394–7.
[88] Maung AA, Fujimi S, Miller ML, et al. Enhanced TLR4 reactivity following injury is mediated by increased p38 activation. J Leukoc Biol 2005;78(2):565–73.
[89] Murphy TJ, Paterson HM, Kriynovich S, et al. Linking the "two-hit" response following injury to enhanced TLR4 reactivity. J Leukoc Biol 2005;77(1):16–23.
[90] Murphy TJ, Paterson HM, Mannick JA, et al. Injury, sepsis, and the regulation of Toll-like receptor responses. J Leukoc Biol 2004;75(3):400–7.

ELSEVIER SAUNDERS

Anesthesiology Clin N Am
24 (2006) 279–297

ANESTHESIOLOGY
CLINICS OF
NORTH AMERICA

Non-pharmacologic Prevention of Surgical Wound Infection

Daniel I. Sessler, MD

*Department of Outcomes Research, the Cleveland Clinic, 9500 Euclid Avenue, E30,
Cleveland, OH 44195, USA*

Wound infections are serious and relatively common postoperative complications. They are generally detected 5 to 9 days after surgery and are usually attributed, even by surgeons, to poor surgical technique or failure to maintain sterility. However, it has been known for decades that all wounds become contaminated, often by bacteria from the skin or within the patient, and that it is host defense mechanisms that prevent most contamination from developing into clinical infections. Host defense is especially important during the initial hours following contamination, the immediate postoperative period.

As might thus be expected, factors that improve host defense reduce infection risk. Many of these are under the direct control of anesthesiologists and are at least as important as the appropriate use of prophylactic antibiotics, which halve infection risk [1]. This article reviews non-pharmacologic methods of reducing infection risk, and emphasizes methods available to anesthesiologists.

This article was supported by NIH Grant GM 061655 (Bethesda, MD), the Gheens Foundation (Louisville, KY), the Joseph Drown Foundation (Los Angeles, CA), and the Commonwealth of Kentucky Research Challenge Trust Fund (Louisville, KY).

E-mail address: sessler@louisville.edu

doi:10.1016/j.atc.2006.01.005 *anesthesiology.theclinics.com*

Background

Wound infections are among the most common serious complications of anesthesia and surgery [2–4]. For example, a study by the Center for Disease Control and Prevention (CDC) reports that the wound infection risk in patients who undergo colon surgery ranges from 9% to 27%, and depends on the duration of surgery, degree of contamination of the wound, and number of underlying diseases [5]. On average, the wound infection rate after a colon resection procedure that lasts longer than 2 hours is reported to be about 15% in most hospitals [5]. More recent values are somewhat lower, but the risk of infection remains distressingly high.

The morbidity (and related cost) associated with surgical infections is considerable; estimates of prolonged hospitalization vary from 5 to 20 days per infection [2,5,6]. Moreover, after-hospital costs are higher because patients who have experienced wound infections are usually discharged before the wound closes entirely and, therefore, require dressing changes two to three times daily. The required supplies are costly, and home-nursing visits may be necessary. Despite the substantial reduction in wound infection rates that result from the universal implementation of sterile technique and prophylactic antibiotics, the incidence of perioperative wound infections remains so high, and so costly, that interventions which produce even small decreases in the infection rate must be considered seriously.

Various factors influence development of wound infections, including (1) character and magnitude of contamination; (2) effects of hemostasis, foreign bodies, and damaged tissues on the local milieu; (3) wound perfusion, which delivers immune components such as oxygen, inflammatory cells, growth factors, cytokines, and nutritional components including amino acids, glucose, and insulin; (4) antibiotic administration; and (5) immune function [7,8]. Non-specific or natural immunity is the most important host defense after acute bacterial contamination, particularly when battling the most common surgical pathogens, including S. Aureus, Klebsiella, E coli, Candida, and Enterococcus [2,3]. Non-specific immune responses include opsonization of bacteria, granulocyte demargination, diapedesis, phagocytosis, and both oxygen-dependent and non-oxidative bacterial killing [9]. Among these, oxidative killing by neutrophils dominates.

The first few hours after bacterial contamination constitute a decisive period during which infection is established [10]. The effects of antibiotic administration and of hypoperfusion are especially important during this period. For example, antibiotics limit infection when given within 3 hours of bacterial inoculation but are ineffective when given more than 3 hours after inoculation [7,11]. Similarly, wound hypoperfusion (achieved by epinephrine infiltration or dehydration shock) aggravates test infections when induced up to 2.5 hours after the inoculation, but has no effect when induced later [10]. Techniques to improve resistance to surgical wound infections are most likely to succeed if implemented during the decisive period. It is because the decisive period is so important that interventions restricted to the perioperative period influence wound infection risk, even though infections are usually detected clinically 5–10 days after surgery.

Maintaining normothermia

Perioperative thermal homeostasis

General [12] and neuraxial [13] anesthesia profoundly impairs thermoregulatory control. Consequently, nearly all unwarmed surgical patients become hypothermic. Hypothermia results initially from a rapid core-to-peripheral redistribution of body heat [14,15] and is followed by a linear reduction in core temperature which results from heat loss that exceeds heat production. Even mild perioperative hypothermia has been causally linked to numerous severe complications including increased blood loss [16] and transfusion requirement [17], morbid myocardial outcomes [18], prolonged post-anesthetic recovery [19] and hospitalization [6], negative nitrogen balance [20], post-anesthetic shivering [21–23], and thermal discomfort [24]. Hypothermia also increases the risk of surgical wound infection.

Hypothermia reduces host defense

Hypothermia may facilitate perioperative wound infections in two ways. First, sufficient intraoperative hypothermia triggers thermoregulatory vasoconstriction [25,26]. Furthermore, vasoconstriction during recovery is universal in hypothermic patients because brain anesthetic concentration decreases rapidly, which facilitates re-emergence of thermoregulatory responses [27]. Thermoregulatory vasoconstriction decreases subcutaneous oxygen tension in humans [28], and the risk of wound infection correlates with subcutaneous oxygen tension [29,30].

Second, considerable evidence indicates that mild core hypothermia directly impairs immune function including T-cell-mediated antibody production [31,32] and non-specific oxidative bacterial killing by neutrophils [8]. Bacterial killing by neutrophils is apparently reduced as temperature decreases from 41°C to 26°C [33,34], although in vitro results depend critically on the model used [35]. Decreased killing results at least in part because production of oxygen and nitroso free radicals is oxygen-dependent within the range of oxygen partial pressures that are found in wounds [36,37].

Patients who have an initial postoperative temperature near 34.5°C—a typical core temperature in unwarmed patients who undergo major surgery [25,26,38]—require several hours to restore core normothermia. Bacterial fixation (ie, the conversion of contamination into an infection), will typically occur when unwarmed patients remain hypothermic. Perioperative hypothermia may contribute to surgical wound infections even though the infections are not usually detected until days after surgery. In contrast, it is unlikely that exaggerated bacterial growth aggravates infections in hypothermic patients because the small differences among in vitro growth rates within the tested temperature range would decrease bacterial growth during hypothermia [39].

Normothermia reduces infection risk

Taken together, these in vitro results suggest that hypothermia may directly impair neutrophil function, or impair it indirectly by triggering subcutaneous vasoconstriction and subsequent tissue hypoxia. Consistent with this theory, mild hypothermia reduces resistance to test infections in animals [40,41]. More importantly, 1.9°C core hypothermia (core temperature of 34.7°C) triples the incidence of surgical wound infection after colon resection [6]. These infections were clinically important as indicated by the fact that infected patients, on average, were hospitalized 1 week longer than the uninfected patients.

A subsequent, uncontrolled, retrospective trial failed to identify a correlation between temperature and infection [42]. This study, though, suffered such serious methodological flaws that it is difficult to interpret [43]. In contrast, a subsequent randomized trial confirmed that both local and systemic warming reduces infection risk—although this may be the only thermoregulatory trial ever published in which core temperature is not reported [44].

Interestingly, hypothermia also increases the duration of hospitalization by 20% even when infected patients are excluded from the analysis—apparently because healing per se was significantly impaired (Table 1) [6]. This result is consistent with studies by Carli and colleagues [6] which showed that mild hypothermia aggravates postoperative protein wasting [20] and mild hypothermia reduces collagen deposition (scar formation).

Excluding brain injury, the major causes of morbidity and mortality in trauma patients are coagulopathy and infection. Since both coagulation [16,17] and resistance to infection [6,44] are profoundly influenced by hypothermia, it is not surprising that outcome would be improved in normothermic trauma patients [45]. The difficulty with this study, however, is that it is a retrospective analysis. This is a grave limitation because the most seriously injured patients are likely to become the most hypothermic. It is difficult to be sure that adverse outcomes result from hypothermia per se rather than underlying injury. Nonetheless, the result is consistent with known effects of hypothermia.

Table 1
Maintaining perioperative normothermia reduces wound infection risk and shortens hospitalization

	Normothermic	Hypothermic	P
Number	104	96	
Temperature (°C)	36.6 ± 0.5	34.7 ± 0.6	<.001
Infection (%)	6	19	<.01
Hospitalization (days)	12.1 ± 4.4	14.7 ± 6.5	.001

Supplemental oxygen

Tissue oxygenation

Oxidative killing of pathogenic bacteria by neutrophils is the most important immune defense against surgical pathogens [46]. Oxidative killing depends on the production of bactericidal superoxide radicals from molecular oxygen. The rate of this reaction, catalyzed by the NADPH (nicotinamide adenine dinucleotide phosphate)-linked oxygenase, is PO_2 (partial pressure, oxygen)-dependent. Our studies indicate that neutrophil superoxide production has a Km for oxygen of the NADPH-linked oxygenase of at least 60 mmHg [47]. Consistent with this observation, oxidative killing is oxygen-dependent from 0 mmHg to ≥ 150 mmHg [48].

Inadequate tissue oxygen also impairs tissue repair. Scar formation requires hydroxylation of abundant proline and lysine residues [49]. The prolyl and lysyl hydroxylases that catalyze this reaction depend on the substrate oxygen [49]. The Michaelis constant (Km) for O_2 of prolyl hydroxylase has been variously estimated at 20, 25, and 100 mmHg [50–52]. Even using the most conservative estimate, proline hydroxylation of collagen will be PO_2-dependent through the range of 0 to at least 200 mmHg; 90% of the effect will occur by 90 mmHg. Consistent with this estimate, hydroxyproline deposition is proportional to arterial PO_2 in rabbits [53] and surgical patients [54].

Partial pressure of oxygen in wounds also has a regulatory component [55,56]. For example, it has been known since the 1980s that oxygen regulates angiogenesis [57,58]. Angiogenesis is mediated by micromolar concentrations of H_2O_2 and other reactive oxygen species that activate vascular endothelial growth factor [59,60].

The partial pressure of oxygen in subcutaneous tissues varies widely, even in patients whose arterial hemoglobin is fully saturated. Many factors are known to influence tissue oxygen tension, including systemic and local temperature [28], smoking [61], anemia [62], perioperative fluid management [54], and uncontrolled surgical pain [63]. But as might be expected, one of the most effective (and least expensive) ways to increase tissue oxygenation is to simply augment inspired oxygen concentration (Fig. 1) [29].

Supplemental oxygen reduces infection risk

The concept that oxygen is an antibiotic was developed by Knighton and colleagues [64,65] in a series of in vitro and animal studies in the 1980s. That tissue oxygenation might have a clinically important effect on wound infection risk was first identified by Hopf and coworkers [30]. In an observational study, they found that infection risk was inversely proportional to postoperative tissue oxygenation. As a natural consequence of its observational design, this study was confounded by the possibility that tissue oxygenation was worse in sicker patients who had the largest operations, and therefore the

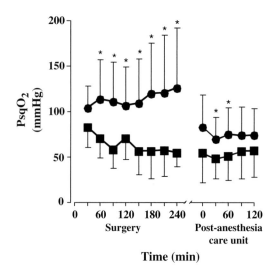

Fig. 1. Subcutaneous oxygen tension, the primary determinant of wound infection risk, during surgery and in the postoperative care unit. Asterisks (*) indicate $P<.01$. Tissue oxygenation was measured in a surrogate wound on the upper arm. Intraoperative tissue oxygen partial pressure was doubled by supplemental oxygen ($FiO_2=80\%$ versus 30%); the effect was less during the postoperative period. Results are expressed as mean $\pm$ SD. PsqO$_2$, tissue oxygen pressure; PACU, post-anesthesia care unit.

greatest infection risk, but that there might not be a causal link between the two observations.

The first randomized trial of supplemental oxygen and wound infection risk by Greif and colleagues [29] involved 500 patients who underwent elective colon resection and who were randomly assigned to an inspired oxygen concentration of 30% (n=246) or 80% (n=254) intraoperatively and for 2 hours after surgery. Wounds were evaluated daily by blinded investigators; both pus and a positive culture were required for diagnosis of infection. Wound scores [66] were 5 ± 9 for the patients who were given 30% oxygen and 3 ± 7 for those who were given 80%, $P=.019$. (All results are expressed as mean ± SD.). There were 13 surgical wound infections in the patients who received 80% oxygen and 28 in those who received 30% ($P=.01$). Supplemental oxygen halved the infection risk.

In contrast, a subsequent report by Pryor and colleagues [67] that included only 160 patients, reported that supplemental oxygen increases the risk of infection. It is worth considering why the results of Pryor and coworkers differ so markedly from those of Greif and coworkers [29]. Pryor and coworkers [67] did not specify the baseline infection rate they used, which makes it impossible to confirm their estimate that 300 patients would be required to detect a 40% reduction in the infection rate. But to have an 80% power to detect the 40% risk reduction that they specified from 25% (our baseline) or from 11% (baseline from Greif and coworkers [29]) would require 540 or 651 patients, respectively; to detect a 40% increase would require 698 or 930 patients, respectively. The study appears to have been underpowered and then stopped after only 160 patients were randomized. The authors specify that 160 patients was an a priori stopping point, although 53.3% of the anticipated sample size is a curious a priori stopping point [68].

A second factor is that in the study by Pryor and colleagues [67], treatment groups were not homogeneous. For example, patients who received 80% oxygen weighed more and were more than twice as likely to have a body-mass index that exceeded 30 kg/m^2. Patients assigned to 80% oxygen also had longer operations, lost significantly more blood, and required significantly more fluid replacement. Furthermore, Pryor and colleagues failed to control many variables believed to influence infection risk, including anesthetic, fluid, antibiotic, and pain management. A third limitation of Pryor's study is that wound infections were determined by retrospective chart review; a review that was apparently conducted by unblinded investigators. This insensitive methodology contrasts markedly with the daily wound evaluations by blinded investigators used by Greif and colleagues. It is possible that these methodological problems contributed to a result that is inconsistent with considerable in vitro, in vivo, and clinical data [69].

The most recent randomized trial of supplemental oxygen by Belda and colleagues [70] involved 300 patients who underwent colon resection and who were randomly assigned to 30% or 80% FiO$_2$ (fraction of inspired oxygen) intra-operatively and 6 hours postoperatively. Blinded investigators diagnosed all wound infections and used CDC criteria. Baseline patient characteristics, anesthetic management, and potential confounding factors were recorded. Wound infection rates were compared by chi-square analysis. Logistic regression was used to assess the contribution of potential confounding factors. Surgical wound infection occurred in 24.4% of the patients who received 30% oxygen, but only 14.9% of those patients who received 80% oxygen ($P = .04$). After adjustment, the relative risk of infection for patients given supplemental oxygen was 0.46 ($P = .04$). Supplemental inspired oxygen reduced wound infection risk by roughly a factor of two.

The most recent trial related to supplemental oxygen and wound infection was conducted by Myles and colleagues [71] and evaluated the effect when supplemental oxygen (80%) was substituted for 70% nitrous oxide in 30% oxygen. Infection risk for the patients given supplemental oxygen was reduced by about 25%. This study differs from previous ones because both nitrous oxide and oxygen concentration varied. It is impossible to determine from the results of Myles and colleagues whether the observed reduction in infection risk resulted from avoidance of nitrous oxide or the beneficial effects of supplemental oxygen.

There are at least three reasons why nitrous oxide might increase infection risk and the authors' hypothesis was that nitrous oxide would reduce host resistance. However, another recent outcome trial by Fleishmann and colleagues [72], specifically compared infection risk in more than 400 patients who were randomly assigned to 65% nitrous oxide or 65% nitrogen; there was no significant difference between the groups. It seems likely, therefore, that reduced infection risk demonstrated in the study by Myles and colleagues [71] results from supplemental oxygen rather than nitrous oxide toxicity per se. This trial provides additional support for the antibiotic effect of supplemental oxygen.

There have now been three randomized trials that specifically evaluate the effect of supplemental oxygen on surgical wound infection. Two trials, a total of 800 patients, each found that 80% FiO_2 reduced infection risk by a factor of two. In contrast, one small study that included only 160 patients and had substantial methodological problems, found just the opposite. Furthermore, an additional study with 2000 patients that found that substituting supplemental oxygen for nitrous oxide significantly reduces infection risk [71]. Because nitrous oxide, per se, does not increase infection risk [72], it is reasonable to consider this study as additional confirmation that supplemental oxygen reduces infection risk. Supplemental oxygen should be provided when practical (Table 2).

In each trial, supplemental oxygen was provided intraoperatively; however, postoperative treatments differed. In the studies by Greif and colleagues [29] and Pryor and colleagues [67] postoperative supplemental oxygen was continued for 2 hours. In contrast, postoperative oxygen was continued for 6 hours in the study by Belda and colleagues [70] and was restricted to the intraoperative period in the study by Myles and coworkers [71]. There is currently no study that directly compares intraoperative oxygen only, with the combination of intraoperative and postoperative oxygen. The extent to which supplemental postoperative oxygen contributes to reduced infection risk thus remains unclear.

Supplemental oxygen is safe

The major complication associated with brief periods of oxygen administration is pulmonary atelectasis. Concern about atelectasis is appropriate because it occurs in up to 85% of patients who undergo lower abdominal surgery and is thought by some to be an important cause of morbidity [73–75]. Two mechanisms contribute to perioperative atelectasis: compression and absorption. Compression results from cephalad displacement of diaphragm, decreased compliance, and reduced functional residual capacity [76]. To some extent, these factors contribute with any anesthetic technique. Absorption, in contrast, is defined by uptake of oxygen from isolated alveoli and results from administration of high oxygen partial pressures. Administration of 100% oxygen, even for a few

Table 2
Randomized trials evaluating the effect of supplemental oxygen on wound infection risk

Source	Number	$FiO_2 = 30\%$ (% infected)	$FiO_2 = 80\%$ (% infected)	P
Greif et al. [29]	500	11	5.0	.01
Pryor et al. [67]	160	11	25.0	.02
Belda et al. [70]	300	24	15.0	.04
Myles et al. [71]	2000	10	7.7	.03

minutes, causes significant postoperative atelectasis by way of this mechanism [74,77].

It is important, though, to distinguish between 100% intraoperative oxygen, which does produce atelectasis, and 80% oxygen, which does not [78]. Akça, and colleagues [69] have shown that 80% perioperative oxygen does not cause atelectasis. Atelectasis was evaluated by computerized tomography the morning after open colon resection. Relatively small amounts of pulmonary atelectasis were observed on the CT scans, and the percentages did not differ significantly in the patients who were given 30% oxygen (2.5 $\pm$ 3.2%) or 80% oxygen (3.0 $\pm$ 1.8%, Fig. 2). Pulmonary function was virtually identical in the two groups.

Hyperoxia causes peripheral vasoconstriction, reduced cardiac output, and slight bradycardia [79], a response that is not sympathetically mediated [80]. In contrast, hypoxia (of a magnitude that is probably common in postoperative patients) is associated with cardiac rhythm disturbances [81] that are prevented by supplemental oxygen [82].

Surgery, anesthesia, cardiopulmonary bypass, and mechanical ventilation each independently impair pulmonary immune defenses [83–85]. Hyperoxia, in contrast, provokes pulmonary expression of inflammatory cytokines, which in turn helps maintain phagocytosis and oxidative killing by alveolar macrophages (Fig. 3) [86]. It is likely that this response helps patients resist pneumonia, but could well become harmful over long periods of time or in the context of other factors promoting pulmonary inflammation.

Operating room fires can result in substantial injury to the patient and health care providers. In United States, there are approximately 2260 reported hospital

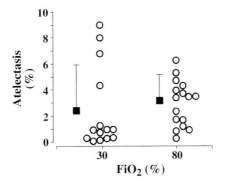

Fig. 2. Relatively small amounts of pulmonary atelectasis were observed on the CT scans, and the percentages did not differ significantly in the patients given 30% oxygen (2.5 $\pm$ 3.2%) or 80% oxygen (3.0 $\pm$ 1.8%). Results are shown for individual patients, along with the group means and SDs. These data provided a 99% chance of detecting a 2% difference in atelectasis volume at an alpha level of 0.05. Poorly aerated regions were also comparable between the groups (9.5 $\pm$ 4.4% in the patients given 30% oxygen versus 10.3 $\pm$ 4.2% in the patients given 80% oxygen). (*From* Akça O, Podolsky A, Eisenhuber E, et al. Comparable postoperative pulmonary atelectasis in patients given 30% or 80% oxygen during and for two hours after colon resection. Anesthesiology 1999;91:997.)

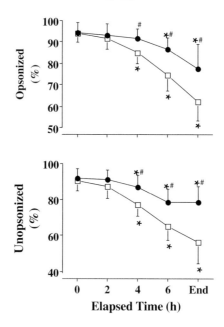

Fig. 3. The fraction of alveolar macrophages that ingest opsonized and non-opsonized particles during anesthesia with 100% (n=30, circles) and 30% (n=30, squares) inspired oxygen. Asterisks (∗) indicate statistically significant differences ($P < .05$) from elapsed time zero in each group; pound signs (#) identify significant differences ($P < .01$) between the two groups. Data are expressed as mean ± SD. (*From* Kotani N, Hashimoto H, Sessler DI, et al. Supplemental intraoperative oxygen augments antimicrobial and proinflammatory responses of alveolar macrophages. Anesthesiology 2000;93(1):22.)

fires per year that result in 1 death and 130 injuries. But among these, fewer than 100 occur in operating rooms and of those, only a small fraction result in injury.

As might be expected, oxygen facilitates ignition of flammable material, such as operating room draping, and speeds propagation of fire once ignited. However, oxygen is normally contained within an anesthesia circuit or well-away from ignition sources such as electrocautery devices. Concerns about operating room fire should thus not normally prevent clinicians from providing supplemental oxygen, and especially not in patients at risk for wound infection because infections are much more common than fires. Even open oxygen (such as provided by nasal prongs) dissipates in less than 10 cm and is unlikely to contribute to fire risk unless the ignition source is immediately proximate to the oxygen source [87].

Surgical site preparation

It is widely believed that hair removal at the operative site reduces contamination and, therefore, infection risk. It remains routine to shave surgical sites. In fact, it is well established that infection rates are lower after clean operations when hair is not removed or when depilatories are used rather than shaving [88]. Furthermore, infection rates are reduced when hair is clipped rather than shaved, even when hair is removed on the day of surgery [89]. The reason, presumably, is that shaving injures skin, and surface bacteria can penetrate. If hair removal at the incision site is considered necessary, it should be removed with clippers during the immediate preoperative period. A corollary is that patients can be warned not to shave their operative sites before surgery, as some shave in an effort to be helpful.

Smoking

Two European studies, published in 1993 and 1996, each showed that smokers have a markedly increased risk of surgical wound infection. These results were not surprising because smoking a single cigarette markedly reduces tissue oxygenation for 1 hour [61]; tissues are nearly always hypoxic in pack-a-day smokers.

Interestingly, though, three subsequent large trials published in 2000 and later, again from Europe, show no relationship between smoking and infection risk (Table 3) [29,70,72]. The reason, presumably, is that smoking is no longer permitted in hospitals. Although smoking obviously produces numerous adverse effects, it no longer appears to be a specific risk factor for development of surgical wound infection.

Glucose control

Patients who have diabetes are at increased risk for all kinds of infectious complications and have two-to-three times the risk of surgical wound infection as patients who do not have diabetes after cardiac operations. For patients who have diabetes and who undergo gastrointestinal or cardiac operations, hyperglycemia (blood glucose exceeding either 200 or 220 mg/dL) is associated with wound infection risk [90,91]. However, it is important to distinguish the long-term peripheral micro-vascular disease of diabetes (which cannot be acutely reversed) with the immediate effects of perioperative hyperglycemia.

Table 3
Smoking and wound infection risk

Source	Year	Non-smokers (% infected/n)	Smokers (% infected/n)	P
Kurz et al. [6]	1996	7/148	22/76	<.001
Greif et al. [29]	2000	8/283	8/122	NS
Fleishmann et al. [72]	2005	16/335	17/81	NS
Belda et al. [70]	2005	22/187	30/46	NS

There are nonetheless reasons to believe that hyperglycemia per se increases infection risk. For example, the risk of surgical site infection for patients who do and do not have diabetes is doubled in cardiac surgical patients when blood glucose exceeds 200 mg/dL in the first 48 hours. Interestingly, half of the observed hyperglycemic episodes occurred in nondiabetic patients [92].

In an observational trial, Furnary and colleagues [93] demonstrated a significant reduction in deep sternal wound infections when perioperative insulin management was switched from subcutaneous administration using a sliding scale to a continuous insulin infusion. Rigorous postoperative glucose control using an aggressive insulin infusion protocol has also been shown to reduce multiple organ failure, sepsis, and mortality in critical care patients [94]. This study, though, is the only published prospective evidence that tight perioperative glucose control improves outcome, and the study focused on cardiac surgical patients who were admitted to a critical care unit. Whether this finding can be extrapolated to other surgical patients remains to be determined.

It is worth noting, though, that glucose control differs from the other interventions discussed in this article. The others are all simple-to-implement, inexpensive, and pose little or no risk. Tight glucose control, in contrast, requires critical care with all the expense that implies, and includes a distinct risk of hypoglycemia. Further study will be required to determine which patients benefit from tight glucose control and whether outcomes improve sufficiently to justify the difficulty and expense.

Potential interventions

Vascular volume

Mild-to-moderate reductions in vascular volume trigger peripheral vasoconstriction to maintain nearly normal blood pressure. However, well-maintained arterial pressure and central organ perfusion comes at the expense of peripheral perfusion, which can be reduced substantially by even small volume deficits. Blood pressure (and urine output) is thus a poor indicator of peripheral perfusion [95].

As might thus be expected, peripheral perfusion and oxygenation were better in surgical patients who were given 16–18 mL $\cdot$ kg$^{-1} \cdot$ h^{-1} than in those who were given 8 mL $\cdot$ kg$^{-1} \cdot$ h^{-1}. The tissue oxygen tension was greater in the high-volume group in both the intraoperative (81 $\pm$ 26 mmHg versus 67 $\pm$ 18 mmHg, $P = .03$) and postoperative periods (77 $\pm$ 26 mmHg versus 59 $\pm$ 15 mmHg, $P = .03$). These results suggest that providing supplemental fluid might reduce infection risk. There is also evidence that titrating perioperative hydration to tissue oxygenation results in more fluid administration and better wound healing [96].

Unfortunately, the results of a subsequent clinical outcome study were less encouraging [97]. Patients who underwent open colon resection were randomly assigned to small- $(8 \ mL \cdot kg^{-1} \cdot h^{-1})$ or large-volume $(16{-}18 \ mL \cdot kg^{-1} \cdot h^{-1})$ fluid management. Infection rates were nearly identical and the study was stopped on a futility basis after about 250 patients were enrolled. It is important to recognize, though, that this study was underpowered and a clinically important effect of fluid management on infection risk remains possible. Other studies identify either improved [98,99] or worsened [100] composite complication rates for patients who were given larger fluid volumes. It is thus unclear from the available literature how fluids should be managed to minimize infection risk. Furthermore, the results are likely to vary as a function of type of surgery, type of fluid, or by dosing scheme (ie, goal-directed versus mL/kg).

Pain relief

Postoperative pain provokes an autonomic response that markedly increases adrenergic nerve activity and plasma catecholamine concentrations [101]. A consequence is arteriolar vasoconstriction. Reduced peripheral perfusion, in turn, would be expected to decrease tissue oxygen partial pressure.

In fact, this theory was confirmed by Akça and colleagues [63] who showed that tissue oxygen partial pressures were 25 mmHg greater in patients who had knee arthroplasty when their pain was aggressively treated (Fig. 4). Whether this translates into lower infection risk has yet to be demonstrated, although a 25-mm increase is probably clinically important [30]. Of course, patients deserve adequate analgesia even if pain relief proves not to reduce infection risk.

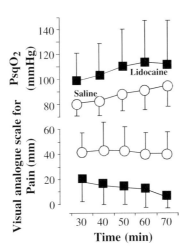

Fig. 4. A study of pain scores and tissue oxygenation in patients who were given intra-articular lidocaine (*squares*) or saline (*circles*). Pain scores, on a 100-mm visual-analog scale, were much larger in patients given saline, and their tissue oxygen partial pressures averaged 25 mmHg less. All values differed significantly between the two groups; data are presented as mean ± SD. VAS, visual analogue scale. (*Reprinted from* Akça O, Melischek M, Scheck T, et al. Postoperative pain and subcutaneous oxygen tension. Lancet 1999;354:41, Copyright (1999), with permission.)

Hypercapnia

The primary determinants of tissue oxygen availability are arterial oxygen content, cardiac output, and local perfusion [102–104]. An important, but often overlooked, influence on cardiac output is arterial carbon dioxide partial pressure [105]. For example, hyperventilation and hypocapnia decrease cardiac output, which in turn decreases blood flow and oxygen tension in brain and splanchnic organs [106–108]. Hypocapnia also shifts the oxyhemoglobin curve leftward and restricts oxygen unloading at the tissue level.

Hypercapnia, in contrast, increases cardiac output, apparently by way of sympathetic nervous system activation, and also improves oxygen extraction. Consequently, hypercapnia increases oxygen availability to tissue [109]. Because hypercapnia during cardiopulmonary bypass does increase tissue oxygenation (O. Akça, et al., unpublished data, 2005), the increase observed in volunteers and routine surgical patients presumably results largely from an increase in cardiac output, rather than primary vasodilation per se.

Hypercapnia also causes a complex interaction between altered cardiac output, hypoxic pulmonary vasoconstriction, and intrapulmonary shunt, which results in a net increase in PaO_2 (partial pressure of oxygen in arterial blood) at a given inspired oxygen concentration [110]. But even at a given PaO_2, there is a linear relationship between arterial carbon dioxide tension and cardiac output and subcutaneous oxygenation. In fact, each mmHg increase in arterial carbon dioxide resulted in a 0.8 mmHg increase in subcutaneous oxygenation in volunteers [111]. The increase was even more impressive in surgical patients: subcutaneous oxygenation increased from 63 ± 14 at a $PaCO_2$ of 30 mmHg to 89 ± 19 at a $PaCO_2$ of 45 mmHg (Fig. 5) [112]. These data suggest that main-

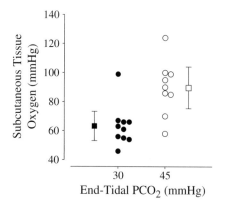

Fig. 5. A study of subcutaneous tissue oxygen as a function of end-tidal PCO_2 in patients who underwent major surgery. Measurements were made on the lateral aspect of the upper arm with a polargraphic electrode system. The mean oxygen tension in the group given 45 mmHg CO_2 was significantly greater ($P = .014$) than it was in the group given 30 mmHg CO_2. Results are presented as mean ± SD. (*From* Akça O, Liem E, Suleman MI, et al. Effect of intra-operative end-tidal carbon dioxide partial pressure on tissue oxygenation. Anaesthesia 2003;58(6):539.)

taining slight hypercapnia, a simple and inexpensive maneuver, may reduce infection risk. This theory, however, has yet to be confirmed.

Summary

Surgical site infections are among the most common serious perioperative complications. Infections are established during a decisive period that lasts a few hours after contamination. Adequacy of host immune defenses is the primary factor that determines whether inevitably wound contamination progresses into a clinical infection. As it turns out, many determinants of infection risk are under the direct control of anesthesiologists; factors that are at least as important as prophylactic antibiotics.

Major outcome studies demonstrate that the risk of surgical wound infection is reduced threefold simply by keeping patients normothermic. Infection risk is reduced by an additional factor of two by if supplemental oxygen is provided (80% versus 30%) during surgery and for the initial hours after surgery. The contribution, if any, of other factors including, tight glucose control, fluid management, and mild hypercapnia have yet to be suitably tested.

References

[1] Platt R, Zaleznik DF, Hopkins CC, et al. Perioperative antibiotic prophylaxis for herniorrhaphy and breast surgery. N Engl J Med 1990;322(3):153–60.

[2] Bremmelgaard A, Raahave D, Beir-Holgersen R, et al. Computer-aided surveillance of surgical infections and identification of risk factors. J Hosp Infect 1989;13:1–18.

[3] Coles B, van Heerden JA, Keys TF, et al. Incidence of wound infection for common general surgical procedures. Surg Gynecol Obstet 1982;154:557–60.

[4] Polk HC, Simpson CJ, Simmons BP, et al. Guidelines for prevention of surgical wound infection. Arch Surg 1983;118:S1213–7.

[5] Haley RW, Culver DH, Morgan WM, et al. Identifying patients at high risk of surgical wound infection: a simple multivariate index of patient susceptibility and wound contamination. Am J Epidemiol 1985;121:206–15.

[6] Kurz A, Sessler DI, Lenhardt RA. Study of wound infections and temperature group. Perioperative normothermia to reduce the incidence of surgical-wound infection and shorten hospitalization. N Engl J Med 1996;334:1209–15.

[7] Burke JF. The effective period of preventive antibiotic action in experimental incisions and dermal lesions. Surgery 1961;50:161–8.

[8] Van Oss CJ, Absolam DR, Moore LL, et al. Effect of temperature on the chemotaxis, phagocytic engulfment, digestion and O_2 consumption of human polymorphonuclear leukocytes. J Reticuloendothel Soc 1980;27:561–5.

[9] Benhaim P, Hunt TK. Natural resistance to infection: leukocyte functions. J Burn Care Rehabil 1992;13:287–92.

[10] Miles AA, Miles EM, Burke J. The value and duration of defence reactions of the skin to the primary lodgement of bacteria. Br J Exp Pathol 1957;38(1):79–96.

[11] Classen DC, Evans RS, Pestotnik R, et al. The timing of prophylactic administration of antibiotics and the risk of surgical wound infection. N Engl J Med 1992;326:281–6.

[12] Xiong J, Kurz A, Sessler DI, et al. Isoflurane produces marked and non-linear decreases in the vasoconstriction and shivering thresholds. Anesthesiology 1996;85:240–5.

[13] Ozaki M, Kurz A, Sessler DI, et al. Thermoregulatory thresholds during spinal and epidural anesthesia. Anesthesiology 1994;81:282–8.

[14] Matsukawa T, Sessler DI, Christensen R, et al. Heat flow and distribution during epidural anesthesia. Anesthesiology 1995;83:961–7.

[15] Matsukawa T, Sessler DI, Sessler AM, et al. Heat flow and distribution during induction of general anesthesia. Anesthesiology 1995;82:662–73.

[16] Winkler M, Akça O, Birkenberg B, et al. Aggressive warming reduces blood loss during hip arthroplasty. Anesth Analg 2000;91(4):978–84.

[17] Schmied H, Kurz A, Sessler DI, et al. Mild intraoperative hypothermia increases blood loss and allogeneic transfusion requirements during total hip arthroplasty. Lancet 1996;347:289–92.

[18] Frank SM, Fleisher LA, Breslow MJ, et al. Perioperative maintenance of normothermia reduces the incidence of morbid cardiac events: a randomized clinical trial. JAMA 1997;277:1127–34.

[19] Lenhardt R, Marker E, Goll V, et al. Mild intraoperative hypothermia prolongs postoperative recovery. Anesthesiology 1997;87:1318–23.

[20] Carli F, Emery PW, Freemantle CAJ. Effect of peroperative normothermia on postoperative protein metabolism in elderly patients undergoing hip arthroplasty. Br J Anaesth 1989;63: 276–82.

[21] Alfonsi P, Adam F, Passard A, et al. Nefopam, a non-sedative benzoxazocine analgesic, selectively reduces the shivering threshold. Anesthesiology 2004;100:37–43.

[22] Alfonsi P, Hongnat JM, Lebrault C, et al. The effects of pethidine, fentanyl and lignocaine on postanesthetic shivering. Anaesthesia 1995;50:214–7.

[23] Alfonsi P, Nourredine KE, Adam F, et al. Effect of postoperative skin-surface warming on oxygen consumption and the shivering threshold. Anaesthesia 2003;58(12):1228–34.

[24] Kurz A, Sessler DI, Narzt E, et al. Postoperative hemodynamic and thermoregulatory consequences of intraoperative core hypothermia. J Clin Anesth 1995;7:359–66.

[25] Sessler DI, Olofsson CI, Rubinstein EH. The thermoregulatory threshold in humans during nitrous oxide-fentanyl anesthesia. Anesthesiology 1988;69:357–64.

[26] Sessler DI, Olofsson CI, Rubinstein EH, et al. The thermoregulatory threshold in humans during halothane anesthesia. Anesthesiology 1988;68:836–42.

[27] Sessler DI, Rubinstein EH, Moayeri A. Physiological responses to mild perianesthetic hypothermia in humans. Anesthesiology 1991;75:594–610.

[28] Sheffield CW, Sessler DI, Hopf HW, et al. Centrally and locally mediated thermoregulatory responses alter subcutaneous oxygen tension. Wound Rep Reg 1997;4:339–45.

[29] Greif R, Akça O, Horn E-P, et al. Outcomes Research™ Group. Supplemental perioperative oxygen to reduce the incidence of surgical wound infection. N Engl J Med 2000;342:161–7.

[30] Hopf HW, Hunt TK, West JM, et al. Wound tissue oxygen tension predicts the risk of wound infection in surgical patients. Arch Surg 1997;132(9):997–1004 [discussion 1005].

[31] Farkas LG, Bannantyne RM, James JS, et al. Effect of two different climates on severely burned rats infected with pseudomonas aeruginosa. Eur Surg Res 1974;6:295–300.

[32] Saririan K, Nickerson DA. Enhancement of murine in vitro antibody formation by hyperthermia. Cell Immunol 1982;74:306–12.

[33] Leijh CJ, Van den Barselaar MT, Van Zwet TL, et al. Kinetics of phagocytosis of staphylococcus aureus and escherichia coli by human granulocytes. Immunology 1979;37:453–65.

[34] Wenisch C, Narzt E, Sessler DI, et al. Mild intraoperative hypothermia reduces production of reactive oxygen intermediates by polymorphonuclear leukocytes. Anesth Analg 1996;82(4): 810–6.

[35] Frohlich D, Wittmann S, Rothe G, et al. Mild hyperthermia down-regulates receptor-dependent neutrophil function. Anesth Analg 2004;99(1):284–92.

[36] Hohn DC, MacKay RD, Halliday B, et al. The effect of oxygen tension on the microbicidal function of leukocytes in wound and in vitro. Surg Forum 1976;27:18–20.

[37] Mader JT. Phagocytic killing and hyperbaric oxygen: antibacterial mechanisms. HBO Reviews 1982;2:37–49.

[38] Kurz A, Sessler DI, Narzt E, et al. Morphometric influences on intraoperative core temperature changes. Anesth Analg 1995;80:562–7.

[39] Mackowisk PA. Direct effects of hyperthermia on pathogenic microorganisms: teleologic implications with regard to fever. Rev Infect Dis 1981;3:508–20.

[40] Sheffield CW, Sessler DI, Hunt TK. Mild hypothermia during isoflurane anesthesia decreases resistance to E. Coli dermal infection in guinea pigs. Acta Anaesthesiol Scand 1994;38:201–5.

[41] Sheffield CW, Sessler DI, Hunt TK, et al. Mild hypothermia during halothane anesthesia decreases resistance to S. Aureus dermal infection in guinea pigs. Wound Rep Reg 1994;2:48–56.

[42] Barone JE, Tucker JB, Cecere J, et al. Hypothermia does not result in more complications after colon surgery. Am Surg 1999;65:356–9.

[43] Sessler DI, Kurz A, Lenhardt R. Hypothermia reduces resistance to surgical wound infections [letter]. Am Surg 1999;65(12):1193–6.

[44] Melling AC, Ali B, Scott EM, et al. Effects of preoperative warming on the incidence of wound infection after clean surgery: a randomised controlled trial. Lancet 2001;358(9285):876–80.

[45] Jurkovich GJ, Greiser WB, Luterman A, et al. Hypothermia in trauma victims: an ominous predictor of survival. J Trauma 1987;27:1019–24.

[46] Babior BM. Oxygen-dependent microbial killing by phagocytes. N Engl J Med 1978;298:659–68.

[47] Allen DB, Maguire JJ, Mahdavian M, et al. Wound hypoxia and acidosis limit neutrophil bacterial killing mechansims. Arch Surg 1997;132:991–6.

[48] Togawa T, Nemoto T, Yamazaki T, et al. A modified internal temperature measurement device. Med Biol Eng 1976;14:361–4.

[49] Prockop DJ, Kivirikko KI, Tuderman L, et al. The biosynthesis of collagen and its disorders: part one. N Engl J Med 1979;301:13–23.

[50] De Jong L, Kemp A. Stoichiometry and kinetics of the prolyl 4-hydroxylase partial reaction. Biochim Biophys Acta 1984;787:105–11.

[51] Hutton JJ, Tappel AL, Udenfriend S. Cofactor and substrate requirements of collagen proline hydroxylase. Arch Biochem Biophys 1967;118:231–40.

[52] Myllyla R, Tuderman L, Kivirikko K. Mechanism of the prolyl hydroxylase reaction 2: kinetic analysis of the reaction sequence. Eur J Biochem 1977;80:349–57.

[53] Goodson WH, Hunt TK. Development of a new miniature method for the study of wound healing in human subjects. J Surg Res 1982;33:394–401.

[54] Jönsson K, Jensen JA, Goodson WH, et al. Tissue oxygenation, anemia, and perfusion in relation to wound healing in surgical patients. Ann Surg 1991;214:605–13.

[55] Gordillo GM, Sen CK. Revisiting the essential role of oxygen in wound healing. Am J Surg 2003;186(3):259–63.

[56] Davidson JD, Mustoe TA. Oxygen in wound healing: more than a nutrient. Wound Repair Regen 2001;9(3):175–7.

[57] Knighton DR, Hunt TK, Scheuenstuhl H, et al. Oxygen regulates the expression of angiogenesis factor by macrophages. Science 1983;221:1283–5.

[58] Knighton DR, Silver IA, Hunt TK. Regulation of wound-healing angiogenesis: effect of oxygen gradients and inspired oxygen concentration. Surgery 1981;90:262–70.

[59] Sen CK, Khanna S, Babior BM, et al. Oxidant-induced vascular endothelial growth factor expression in human keratinocytes and cutaneous wound healing. J Biol Chem 2002;277(36):33284–90.

[60] Cho M, Hunt TK, Hussain MZ. Hydrogen peroxide stimulates macrophage vascular endothelial growth factor release. Am J Physiol Heart Circ Physiol 2001;280(5):H2357–63.

[61] Jensen JA, Goodson WH, Hopf HW, et al. Cigarette smoking decreases tissue oxygen. Arch Surg 1991;126:1131–4.

[62] Gosain A, Rabin J, Reymond JP, et al. Tissue oxygen tension and other indicators of blood loss or organ perfusion during graded hemorrhage. Surgery 1991;109:523–32.

[63] Akça O, Melischek M, Scheck T, et al. Postoperative pain and subcutaneous oxygen tension. Lancet 1999;354:41–2.

[64] Knighton DR, Fiegel VD, Halverson T, et al. Oxygen as an antibiotic. the effect of inspired oxygen on bacterial clearance. Arch Surg 1990;125(1):97–100.

[65] Knighton DR, Halliday B, Hunt TK. Oxygen as an antibiotic: the effect of inspired oxygen on infection. Arch Surg 1984;119:199–204.

[66] Byrne DJ, Malek MM, Davey PG, et al. Postoperative wound scoring. Biomed Pharmacother 1989;43:669–73.

[67] Pryor KO, Fahey 3rd TJ, Lien CA, et al. Surgical site infection and the routine use of peri-operative hyperoxia in a general surgical population: a randomized controlled trial. JAMA 2004;291(1):79–87.

[68] Greif R, Sessler DI. Supplemental oxygen and risk of surgical site infection [letter]. JAMA 2004;291(16):1957 [author reply 1958–9].

[69] Akca O, Sessler DI. Supplemental oxygen and risk of surgical site infection [letter]. JAMA 2004;291(16):1956–7 [author reply 1958–9].

[70] Belda FJ, Aguilera L, Garcia de la Asuncion J, et al. Supplemental perioperative oxygen and the risk of surgical wound infection: a randomized controlled trial. JAMA 2005;294(16): 2035–42.

[71] Myles PS, Leslie K, Silbert B, et al. Evaluation of nitrous oxide in the gas mixture for anesthesia: a randomized controlled trial (the ENIGMA trial) [abstract]. Anesthesiology 2005; 103:A681.

[72] Fleischmann E, Lenhardt R, Kurz A, et al. Nitrous oxide and risk of surgical wound infection: a randomised trial. Lancet 2005;366(9491):1101–7.

[73] Lindberg P, Gunnarsson L, Tokics L, et al. Atelectasis and lung function in the postoperative period. Acta Anaesthesiol Scand 1992;36(6):546–53.

[74] Joyce CJ, Baker AB. Effects of inspired gas composition during anaesthesia for abdominal hysterectomy on postoperative lung volumes. Br J Anaesth 1995;75(4):417–21.

[75] Schwieger I, Gamulin Z, Suter PM. Lung function during anesthesia and respiratory insuf-ficiency in the postoperative period: pysiological and clinical implications. Acta Anaesthesiol Scand 1989;33(7):527–34.

[76] Krayer S, Rehder K, Vettermann J, et al. Position and motion of the human diaphragm during anesthesia-paralysis. Anesthesiology 1989;70(6):891–8.

[77] Rothen HU, Sporre B, Engberg G, et al. Reexpansion of atelectasis during general anaesthesia may have a prolonged effect. Acta Anaesthesiol Scand 1995;39(1):118–25.

[78] Edmark L, Kostova-Aherdan K, Enlund M, et al. Optimal oxygen concentration during in-duction of general anesthesia. Anesthesiology 2003;98(1):28–33.

[79] Lodato RF, Jubran A. Response time, autonomic mediation, and reversibility of hyperoxic bradycardia in conscious dogs. J Appl Physiol 1993;74(2):634–42.

[80] Haque WA, Boehmer J, Clemson BS, et al. Hemodynamic effects of supplemental oxygen administration in congestive heart failure. J Am Coll Cardiol 1996;27(2):353–7.

[81] Rosenberg J, Rasmussen V, von Jessen F, et al. Late postoperative episodic and constant hypoxaemia and associated ECG abnormalities. Br J Anaesth 1990;65(5):684–91.

[82] Stausholm K, Kehlet H, Rosenberg J. Oxygen therapy reduces postoperative tachycardia. Anaesthesia 1995;50(8):737–9.

[83] Kotani N, Hashimoto H, Sawamura D, et al. Expression of genes for pro-inflammatory cytokines in alveolar macrophages during propofol and isoflurane anesthesia. Anesth Analg 1999;89:1250–6.

[84] Kotani N, Hashimoto H, Sessler DI, et al. Intraoperative modulation of alveolar macrophage function during isoflurane and propofol anesthesia. Anesthesiology 1998;89:1125–32.

[85] Kotani N, Hashimoto H, Sessler DI, et al. Cardiopulmonary bypass produces greater pulmo-nary than systemic proinflammatory cytokines. Anesth Analg 2000;90(5):1039–45.

[86] Kotani N, Hashimoto H, Sessler DI, et al. Supplemental intraoperative oxygen augments antimicrobial and proinflammatory responses of alveolar macrophages. Anesthesiology 2000; 93(1):15–25.

[87] Reyes RJ, Smith AA, Mascaro JR, et al. Supplemental oxygen: ensuring its safe delivery during facial surgery. Plast Reconstr Surg 1995;95(5):924–8.

[88] Cruse PJE, Foord R. A five-year prospective study of 23,649 surgical wounds. Arch Surg 1973; 107:206–10.

[89] Ko W, Lazenby WD, Zelano JA, et al. Effects of shaving methods and intraoperative irrigation on suppurative mediastinitis after bypass operations. Ann Thorac Surg 1992;53(2):301–5.

[90] Zerr KJ, Furnary AP, Grunkemeier GL, et al. Glucose control lowers the risk of wound infection in diabetics after open heart operations. Ann Thorac Surg 1997;63(2):356–61.

[91] Pomposelli JJ, Baxter 3rd JK, Babineau TJ, et al. Early postoperative glucose control predicts nosocomial infection rate in diabetic patients. JPEN J Parenter Enteral Nutr 1998;22(2):77–81.

[92] Dellinger EP. Preventing surgical-site infections: the importance of timing and glucose control. Infect Control Hosp Epidemiol 2001;22(10):604–6.

[93] Furnary AP, Zerr KJ, Grunkemeier GL, et al. Continuous intravenous insulin infusion reduces the incidence of deep sternal wound infection in diabetic patients after cardiac surgical procedures. Ann Thorac Surg 1999;67(2):352–60 [discussion 360–2].

[94] van den Berghe G, Wouters P, Weekers F, et al. Intensive insulin therapy in the surgical intensive care unit. N Engl J Med 2001;345(19):1359–67.

[95] Jonsson K, Jensen JA, Goodson 3rd WH, et al. Assessment of perfusion in postoperative patients using tissue oxygen measurements. Br J Surg 1987;74(4):263–7.

[96] Hartmann M, Jonsson K, Zederfeldt B. Effect of tissue perfusion and oxygenation on accumulation of collagen in healing wounds. Randomized study in patients after major abdominal operations. Eur J Surg 1992;158(10):521–6.

[97] Kabon B, Akca O, Taguchi A, et al. Supplemental intravenous crystalloid administration does not reduce the risk of surgical wound infection. Anesth Analg 2005;101(5):1546–53.

[98] Gan TJ, Soppitt A, Maroof M, et al. Goal-directed intraoperative fluid administration reduces length of hospital stay after major surgery. Anesthesiology 2002;97(4):820–6.

[99] Holte K, Klarskov B, Christensen DS, et al. Liberal versus restrictive fluid administration to improve recovery after laparoscopic cholecystectomy: a randomized, double-blind study. Ann Surg 2004;240(5):892–9.

[100] Brandstrup B, Tonnesen H, Beier-Holgersen R, et al. Effects of intravenous fluid restriction on postoperative complications: comparison of two perioperative fluid regimens: a randomized assessor-blinded multicenter trial. Ann Surg 2003;238(5):641–8.

[101] Halter JB, Pflug AE, Porte D. Mechanism of plasma catecholamine increases during surgical stress in man. J Clin Endocrin Metab 1977;45:936–44.

[102] Rooth G, Hedstrand U, Tyden H, et al. The validity of transcutaneous oxygen tension method in adults. Crit Care Med 1976;4:162–5.

[103] Tremper K, Shoemaker W. Transcutaneous oxygen monitoring of critically ill adults with, and without low flow shock. Crit Care Med 1981;9:706–9.

[104] Tremper K, Waxman K, Shoemaker W. Effects of hypoxia and shock on transcutaneous PO2 values in dogs. Crit Care Med 1979;7:526–31.

[105] Laffey JG, Kavanagh BP. Carbon dioxide and the critically ill–too little of a good thing? Lancet 1999;354(9186):1283–6.

[106] Barker S, Hyatt J, Clarke C, et al. Hyperventilation reduces transcutaneous oxygen tension and skin blood flow. Anesthesiology 1991;75:619–24.

[107] Domino K, Lu Y, Einstein B, et al. Hypocapnia worsens arterial blood oxygenation and increases VA/Q heterogeneity in canine pulmonary edema. Anesthesiology 1993;78(1):91–9.

[108] Gustaffson U, Sjoberg F, Lewis D, et al. The effect of hypocapnia on skeletal muscle microcirculatory blood flow, oxygenation, and pH. Int J Microcirc Clin Exp 1993;12(2):131–41.

[109] Mas A, Saura P, Joseph D, et al. Effects of acute moderate changes in $PaCO_2$ on global hemodynamics and gastric perfusion. Crit Care Med 2000;28(2):360–5.

[110] Hickling K, Joyce C. Permissive hypercapnia in ARDS and its effects on tissue oxygenation. Acta Anaesthesiol Scand 1995;107:201–8.

[111] Akça O, Doufas AG, Morioka N, et al. Hypercapnia improves tissue oxygenation. Anesthesiology 2002;97(4):801–6

[112] Akça O, Liem E, Suleman MI, et al. Effect of intra-operative end-tidal carbon dioxide partial pressure on tissue oxygenation. Anaesthesia 2003;58(6):536–42.

ELSEVIER
SAUNDERS

Anesthesiology Clin N Am
24 (2006) 299–323

ANESTHESIOLOGY
CLINICS OF
NORTH AMERICA

Bioecologic Control of Inflammation and Infection in Critical Illness

Stig Bengmark, MD, PhD*

*Institute of Hepatology, University College London Medical School, 69-75 Chenies Mews,
London WC1E 6HX, UK*

Advanced surgical and medical treatments and medical and surgical emergencies are, despite some breathtaking advances in medical-pharmaceutical and surgical treatment, still affected by an unacceptably high rate of morbidity and mortality. Worse, the rate of both morbidity and mortality in critical illness (CI) is quickly increasing and has done so for several decades. With a documented rate increase of 1.5% per year, the rate has the potential to double within the coming 50 to 60 years. Sepsis is the most common medical and surgical complication, estimated in the United States alone to affect as many as 751,000 [1,2] patients and cause the deaths of approximately 215,000 patients (29%) annually [2,3], which makes sepsis the tenth most common cause of death in the country [4].

Presently available treatment options such as antibiotics and antagonists and inhibitors of individual proinflammatory cytokines have not met the early, high expectations. Instead, these treatments have often precipitated new complications and new morbidities. Selective bowel decontamination (eg, parallel parenteral and topical application of a handful of powerful antibiotics) is no longer a treatment option. After more than 30 years of dedicated efforts to combat sepsis by the use of various combinations of antibiotics and more than 30 randomized clinical trials, we seem ready to conclude that the vigorous use of antibiotics, despite some observations of a modest decrease in incidence of chest infections, does not significantly reduce mortality in critically ill patients [5]. Two recent multicenter studies document no effects from antibiotic treatment in severe acute pancreatitis [6,7]. Cytokine inhibitors have most often failed when used in acute disease and critical illness [8], but the reported effects in chronic illnesses are somewhat more promising [9]. Still, side effects and price constitute important obstacles, especially when it comes to long-term treatments.

---

* 185 Barrier Point Road, Royal Docks, London E16 2SE, UK.
E-mail address: s.bengmark@ucl.ac.uk

0889-8537/06/$ – see front matter © 2006 Elsevier Inc. All rights reserved.
doi:10.1016/j.atc.2006.01.002   *anesthesiology.theclinics.com*

A Tsunami of chronic illness

It is well known that the majority of individuals who end up in ICUs are elderly and have one or several chronic illnesses and other signs of reduced resistance to disease. The Katrina of critical illness is strongly associated with a tsunami of chronic diseases (ChDs) affecting the entire world. The World Health Organization estimates that 46% of the global disease burden and 59% of global mortality is caused by ChDs. Thirty-five million individuals die each year from chronic diseases, and this number is increasing steadily [10]. This increase, which seems to have begun at the time of the Industrial Revolution (eg, in the middle of the 1850s), was relatively slow during the first 100 years but has, in recent decades, obtained epidemic proportions. Circumstantial evidence supports the association of ChDs with modern life style factors such as stress, lack of exercise, abuse of tobacco and alcohol, and a transition from natural unprocessed foods to processed, calorie-condensed, and heat-treated foods. The association between the reduced intake of plant fibers, plant antioxidants, increased consumption of dairy products, refined sugars and starch products, and increases in both ChDs and CI is obvious. The per capita consumption of refined sugar has increased from approximately 1 lb/person/y in 1850 to approximately 100 lbs/person/y in the year 2000, and the per cow milk production has increased from 2 to 50 quarts/d. Dairy products, especially milk (mostly from pregnant cows) are rich in proinflammatory molecules, hormones such as estrogens, and growth factors such as insulin-like growth factor-I. Heating up makes it also rich in advanced glycation end (AGEs) products, which also are proinflammatory molecules. Consumption of bovine milk has been shown to release inflammatory mediators, increase intestinal permeability, and induce leakage of molecules such as albumin and hyaluronan. This information is important because many enteral nutrition solutions are based on milk powder. Bread, especially from gluten-containing grains, is also rich in molecules with documented proinflammatory effects [11–13].

The fastest increase of ChDs occurs among people who are poor and have a low degree of education, and this trend is today most pronounced in the third world. We seem to export these diseases together with our cultural, political, and religious values and with our enormous surplus of cheap agricultural products, grains, especially wheat, and dairy products, milk powder, and butter. Little consideration is given to the fact that a large proportion of individuals in these parts of the world is gluten- or lactose-intolerant or to the detrimental effect of such a policy on the local production of health-promoting fresh fruits and vegetables.

Premorbid health determines outcome

Signs of a failing immune system predate the onset of acute, critical illness in the majority of patients. Approximately half of the patients affected by sepsis are in the age group of >65 years, and 48% of the patients are neutropenic [14,15]. Both flora and lining mucosal cells (especially of the intestine) have endocrine functions and are producing and responding to hormones. The gastrointestinal (GI) tract contains 100 million neurons, which is equal to the number of neurons in the spinal cord, distributed through all layers of the GI tract [16] and exerting strong effects on both immune cells and flora, thereby affecting homeostasis of the immune system and resistance to disease. A series of experiments have demonstrated an increase of up to 100,000 times (5 orders of magnitude) in the growth of gram-negative bacteria exposed to noradrenaline [17], which explains a relatively old observation of significantly higher blood levels of noradrenaline and adrenaline in patients who develop severe septic conditions compared with patients who have an uncomplicated postoperative course [18]. The luminal release of noradrenaline strongly induces an increased virulence of luminal bacteria [19], and much evidence suggests that under conditions of stress, potentially pathogenic microorganisms (PPMs) that are normally indolent colonizers change their phenotypes and become life-threatening pathogens [20].

Our knowledge about the innate immune system and its function and our understanding of resistance to disease has increased significantly over the last 10 to 15 years. Solid evidence suggests that the outcome after larger surgical operations as well as in medical emergencies is intimately associated with pre-morbid health and strength of the immune system and is reflected by the speed and depth of functional deterioration during the few hours after trauma. A recent study suggests four important outcome variables in severe acute pancreatitis, high age, chronic health status, need for mechanical ventilation, and increase in serum creatinine during the first 60 to 72 hours, are strongly associated with poor outcome [21]. An alternative prognostic system based on body mass index, age, chest radiography, and oxygen saturation has also been suggested [22].

An immune dysfunction

Modern man is richly exposed to chemicals. The effects on immune functions of pharmaceuticals is often unknown and unappreciated because federal agencies do not regularly require testing new drugs for immune effects. The evidence from experimental studies, however, allows the assumption that a large proportion of the pharmaceuticals used in the ICUs have depressive effects on the immune function. For example, many of the drugs used are shown to derange macrophage functions and bactericidal efficacy and the production and secretion of cytokines. Supplying antibiotics (150 mg/kg body weight of mezlocillin) results in the significant suppression of essential macrophage functions, demonstrated in studies of chemiluminescent response, chemotactic motility, bactericidal and cytostatic ability, and of lymphocyte proliferation [23].

Homeostasis is important for bodily functions and particularly for the immune system and resistance to disease. Chemical substances, depending on dose, can have both stimulatory and inhibitory functions, a phenomenon given the name of chemical hormesis and referred to as the Arndt–Schultz law [24]. A broad range of chemicals has been shown to have immunostimulatory-preventive effects on morbidity in lower doses and immunoinhibitory-disease-inducing effects in larger doses. These effects become more pronounced when the regulatory functions of the gut and liver are bypassed through parenteral administration, a fact largely ignored in the past, when it was believed that parenteral infusion of large amounts of water, electrolytes, and nutrients such as fat and sugar would benefit the patient and improve outcome. Today, it is well known that supplying, especially parenterally, larger amounts of fluid and electrolytes [25–27], fat [28–30], sugar [31,32], and nutrients [33,34] leads to immune dysfunction, reduces resistance to disease, and increases morbidity.

Limited nutrition preserves immunity

Excessive nutrition, parenterally and even enterally, is frequently accompanied by serious, sometimes fatal, metabolic consequences [34] and should be avoided. Total parenteral nutrition (TPN) is rarely, if ever, indicated in perioperative and post-trauma nutrition, at least not during the first 2 weeks after surgery or trauma, as demonstrated in a well-designed randomized study in 300 patients undergoing major general surgery [35]. TPN was provided during a period of up to 15 post-operative days and compared with the infusion of only 1000 to 1500 kcal/d of glucose. The nitrogen loss during the first week was reduced to approximately half in the glucose-supplied group compared with the TPN group, but no differences in morbidity or mortality were observed. Only approximately 20% of the patients who were unable to go back to normal eating within 2 weeks seemed to benefit from TPN. The authors concluded that "overfeeding seemed to be a larger problem than underfeeding." Another somewhat similarly designed study from Memorial-Sloan-Kettering Cancer Center (New York) reaches similar conclusions [36]. One hundred ninety-five patients undergoing resection for upper gastrointestinal malignancies were randomized to either early enteral supplementation with a so-called immunoenhancing diet (a mixture of several nutrients, including Omega-3, L-arginine, and RNA fragments) or only intravenous crystalloid infusions. The daily intake of calories was low in both groups, 1000 and 400 kcal, respectively (eg, 61% and 22%, respectively, of defined goals of 25 kcal/kg/d). No differences in the number of minor, major, or infectious complications or wound infections, mortality, or length of stay (median 11 days for each group) were observed between the groups.

Hyperinflammation

Patients who develop severe septic complication are known to respond to physical and mental stress with an early, exuberant acute or chronic super-inflammation, with signs of exaggerated and prolonged release of proinflammatory cytokines such as interleukin (IL)-6, acute phase proteins such as C-reactive protein, and plasminogen activator inhibitor (PAI)-1 [15]. This reaction is strongly associated with a subsequent severe exacerbation of disease, including acute respiratory distress and multiple organ failure (MOF). Among the changes observed in the over-exuberant acute phase response, often called the nervous phase, are augmented endothelial adhesion of polymorphonuclear (PMN) cells, increased production of intercellular adhesion molecule (ICAM)-1, priming of the PMNs for an oxidative burst, release of proinflammatory platelet activating factor, and associated with this, a delay in PMN apoptosis [37]. Visceral adipocytes are, compared with subcutaneous fat cells, known to secrete much more free fatty acids but also approximately three times as much of IL-6 and PAI-1 per gram tissue, observations that explain well the high risk of both chronic and acute diseases in individuals with visceral obesity [38]. The stress-induced load on organs such as the lung and the liver of these and other proinflammatory and procoagulant molecules can vary by 1000 times or more because the amount of fat in the abdomen can vary from few a milliliters in a lean subject to approximately 6 L in gross obesity [39].

Immunoparesis

Severe trauma, major surgery, and severe sepsis will, in parallel with a significant decrease in lymphocytes, induce a significant increase in circulating and tissue neutrophils. In a study of patients who had undergone severe trauma, Menges and colleagues [40] reported a marked depression of immunity, with a persistent decline in helper T $(T_H)4$ lymphocytes and an elevation of suppressor T $(T_C)8$ lymphocytes. It was suggested that a T_H4/T_C8 lymphocyte cell ratio of <1 is a sign of severe immunosuppression and is a prediction of a complication such as multiple organ dysfunction syndrome, which was verified in patients who had myocardial infarction, acute pancreatitis, and multiple severe trauma, and in oncology ICU patients [41]. Paralleling the decrease in lymphocytes, a significant increase in circulating neutrophils and the accumulation of neutrophils in tissues will occur, often observed and reported in conditions such as shock, sepsis, major trauma, major burns, and severe acute pancreatitis. Accumulating evidence suggests that the tissue infiltration of neutrophils in trauma induces common post-trauma and postoperative dysfunctions such as paralytic ileus [42,43], bone marrow suppression, and endothelial cell dysfunction and results in tissue destruction and organ failure, particularly in lungs [44–46], intestines [47], liver [48], and kidney [49]. Neutrophil infiltration of distant organs [50], especially of the lungs [44], is also a characteristic finding in patients dying of sepsis, and 20 years ago, it was suggested to be a consequence of "generalized auto-destructive inflammation" [50]. The extent of neutrophil infiltration is significantly aggravated by mechanical therapeutic efforts such as handling of the bowels during an operation [42] and ventilation of the lungs [51]. It is also influenced by poor nutritional status, pre-existing immune deficiency, obesity, diabetes and high levels of serum glucose [52], and strongly associated with increased expressions in the body of molecules such as nuclear factor (NF)-κB,

cyclooxygenase (COX)-2, lipoxygenase (LOX), and inducible nitric oxide synthase inhibitor (iNOS) [53,54]. A recent study emphasizes the role of suppressed
apoptosis of circulating neutrophils and the association with increased activation
of NF-κB and reduced activity of caspase-9 and -3 in patients who have clinical
sepsis [55].

The lungs in focus

The most frequently observed and most often severe clinical manifestations of
organ failure are seen in the lungs. In severe acute pancreatitis, the organ systems
most often involved in early (within 24 hours) single-organ failure are pulmonary
(91% and 81%) [56,57]), renal (4.5% and 5%) [56,57], and coagulation (4.5%
and 14%) [56,57]. Extensive neutrophil infiltration of the lungs and also of
other distant organs is a characteristic finding in patients dying of sepsis, and
the degree of oxidative stress and of neutrophil activation and infiltration, especially in the lungs, appears to be the main determining factor of outcome [58].
Acute lung injury is characterized by alveolar capillary endothelial cell injury,
increased capillary permeability and subsequent hypoxia, and an accumulation of
the neutrophil-associated inflammatory products reactive oxygen species (ROS),
proteolytic enzymes, eucosanoid, and various other mediators. Splanchnic hypoperfusion with endothelial cell injury, the increased expression of intercellular
ICAM-1 [59], and serine proteases released by the hypoxic pancreas [60]
mesenteric lymph, transported through the lymphatics and thoracic duct rather
than portal vein [59–61], are in addition to various cytokines [62] suggested to
initiate neutrophil-mediated tissue injuries, particularly in the lungs. Experimental
studies have also shown that post-shock mesenteric lymph will activate the
mechanisms leading to acute lung injury [59] and that the diversion of thoracic
duct lymph will prevent trauma-hemorrhagic shock-induced lung injury [63].

Monitoring immunoparesis

The post-trauma inflammatory response has at least three distinctly different
phases, with significantly different changes in the body and also different nutritional demands, and will require different treatment, including different feeding [64]. Although premorbid health status [65,66] has a strong influence on
outcome, much can still be done especially in the early (nervous) phase (the first
24–36 hours) to reduce the degree of hyperinflammation and limit the extent of
immunoparalysis to occur in the subsequent phase, the immune phase. High
levels of IL-6 and PAI-1 are suggested as prognosticators of outcome, both in
acute conditions after an operation or trauma, myocardial infarction, and pancreatitis, and in semichronic or chronic inflammatory conditions, such as arthritis,
mental depression, or Alzheimer disease. It has been observed in severe acute
pancreatitis that a narrow therapeutic window exists during the first 24 to

36 hours, which should be used to optimize outcome [67]. The effect on outcome of early hyperinflammation was demonstrated in a study in human liver transplantation. All patients who demonstrated a sixfold or higher increase in tumor necrosis factor (TNF)-α and IL-6 during the late phase of the operation developed sepsis during subsequent postoperative days [68].

Shock on admission day is also reported as a strong predictor of outcome, even if adjusted for variables such as degree of hypoxemia and severity scores [69]. Blood glucose levels, especially during the early, nervous phase, are suggested to reflect the extent of stress and degree of inflammation during the nervous phase. Admission levels or preoperative glucose levels are reported to be predictive of subsequent morbidity and mortality in trauma patients [70]. Hyperglycemia, which remains high during subsequent days, is associated with prolonged ventilation, increased rate of infections, length of ICU stay, morbidity, and mortality [71].

The role of HLA-DR

Great interest recently has been given to the expression of HLA-DR as a reliable marker of immunoparesis, and several studies, especially in severe acute pancreatitis, demonstrate a good correlation to increased risk and fatal outcome [72,73]. It is disappointing, however, that the efficacy of HLA-DR seems to reflect mainly the degree of immunoparesis in the immune phase and that the test is less useful when most needed, in the early nervous phase [74–76]. Studies in cardiac surgery patients have found preoperative and immediately postoperative (first 24 hours) HLA-DR levels not to be predictable of increased risk of systemic inflammatory response syndrome (SIRS) and sepsis or infectious complications [77]. In the absence of reliable early markers of poor outcome, it will be interesting to see whether the presence of "sticky neutrophils" before surgery is capable of identifying patients who develop postoperative infections [78]. As suggested by Zahorec [41], the use of the neutrophil/lymphocyte ratio (normal 5.5–8.4, high 18–36, and extreme >36 levels of stress) might also be worth further exploration.

Reducing immunoparesis

The highest priority should be given to early efforts to avoid and minimize treatments that will deepen the subsequent immunoparesis, such as the use of antibiotics, parenteral nutrition, both glucose and macromolecules, stored blood, drains and tubes, and efforts to reduce mechanical manipulation of tissues, both surgical and mechanical ventilation [79,80]. Supplying nutrition enterally must also be performed with care, and nutrition solutions that increase blood glucose levels should be avoided because hyperglycemia is associated with neutrophil dysfunction [81] and significantly increased infection and mortality rates, as demonstrated in trauma patients [82]. Also, commercial enteral nutrition solu-

tions rich in proinflammatory molecules (those containing dairy-derived proinflammatory molecules) should be avoided. In animal experiments, total parenteral solutions and some commercial enteral diets have been shown to activate
iNOS and disrupt the gut barrier function and the intestinal microflora and induce bacterial translocation [83]. Hospital-produced nutrition formulas consisting
of fresh fruits, vegetables (especially legumes), and fish and meat and probably
more suitable for enteral nutrition have, for questionable hygienic and efficiency
reasons, been abandoned at hospitals in the developed world. Controlled clinical
studies comparing the effects of standard nutrition solutions and hospital-made
nutrition solutions on immunity and outcome are most desirable. A recent meta-
analysis based on 20 peer-reviewed articles and more than 13,000 patients reports an average increase of 3.5 times in postoperative infections in surgical
patients receiving allogeneic blood transfusion [84].

Preventing immunoparesis

Stress and acute and chronic phase responses involve numerous molecules and
pathways and affect multiple functions. Most pharmaceutical drugs designed to
prevent inflammation are constructed to specifically block one molecule or pathway, which seems to explain why the success has been and will continue to be
limited, both in acute and chronic inflammatory conditions. The body's acute
phase response possesses numerous pathways, which effectively will bypass phar-
maceutically inhibited functions. Bioecologic control (eg, the use of antioxidants,
anti-inflammatory ω-3 lipid emulsions, bioactive fibers, and probiotic bacteria)
has the advantage of modulating "all pathways" in parallel. The effects of
antioxidants and ω-3 lipid emulsions remain largely unexplored, but significant
modulatory effects on neutrophils and morbidity have been observed in the few
studies thus far [85–87]. Most attempts with antioxidants have been given with
regular vitamins or with glutamine and glutathione. It is important to recognize
that fruit- and vegetable-derived polyphenols of various kinds demonstrate sometimes up to 10 times stronger antioxidative effects. Among these antioxidants
are resveratrol from red wine and peanuts, quercetin from apples and onions, and
curcumin from turmeric, and many others. Curcumin is not only a powerful antioxidant but also a natural, powerful, and totally atoxic inhibitor of NF-κB,
COX-2, LOX, and iNOS; and it has shown strong preventive effects of induced
diseases in several experimental studies and in patients who had acute pancreas
and liver injuries and those who have chronic diseases such as Alzheimer, cancer,
and diabetes [54]. It is important to find out whether these compounds can be tried
in surgical and critically ill patients. Some bioactive fibers and probiotic bacteria
have demonstrated extraordinary efficacy to restore and maintain immunity and
prevent complications. Lactic acid bacteria (LAB) have demonstrated the ability to

- Reduce or eliminate potentially pathogenic microorganisms (PPMs)
- Reduce or eliminate various toxins, mutagens, and carcinogens

- Promote apoptosis
- Synthesize and/or release numerous nutrient; antioxidants, growth, coagulation, and other bioactive compounds
- Modulate the innate and adaptive immune defense mechanisms [88–90]

More recent studies suggest that LAB can

- Promote and maintain GI motility and prevent GI paralysis and post-operative ileus [91–93] and has the ability to inhibit NF-κB activation [94–96]
- Inhibit constitutive synthesis of IL-8 and synthesis and secretion of IL-8 induced by TNF-α [96,97]
- Inhibit COX-2 expression and restore the COX-1/COX-2 ratio [98]

Some of these effects are produced by both live and dead LAB. However, the inhibition of synthesis and secretion of IL-8 are induced by live LAB and not by bacterial lysate, heat-killed, or gamma-irradiated LAB [97]. Immunomodulatory effects are also induced by microbial products, such as butyrate, propionate, pyruvate, and sometimes also by lactate and acetate. Butyrate and propionate for example decrease COX-2 expression with 85% and 72%, respectively, and increase COX-1 expression with 37% and 23%, respectively, effects that cannot be obtained with lactate or acetate [98]. Of great interest in this connection are recent observations by Fink, who observed that supplemented pyruvate is an effective scavenger of ROS and exhibits strong anti-inflammatory effects. Supplemental pyruvate suppresses NF-κB activation, reduces release of NO and proinflammatory cytokines, prevents intestinal translocation, reduces cardiac ischemia, and improves kidney function [99]. Cardio-protective effects have also been reported from the intravenous administration of lyophilized LAB [100].

Lactic acid bacteria prevents neutrophil infiltration and tissue destruction

It was recently demonstrated in experimental animals subjected to cecal ligation and puncture that stress-induced neutrophil infiltration of the lung and subsequent tissue destruction can be prevented effectively by oral supplementation of a synbiotic (pre- and pro-biotics combination) cocktail. A synbiotic formulation of the four LABs in the cocktail, Synbiotic 2000 Forte (Medipharm, Kågeröd, Sweden, and Des Moines, Iowa), administered orally [101] or by sub-cutaneous injection [102] before the trauma, effectively prevented both neutrophil accumulation and tissue destruction in the lungs (Fig. 1). The average neutrophil counts in lung tissue (average of five fields) after enteral administration were: (1) 9.00 ± 0.44 in a mixture of LAB and bioactive fibers; (2) 8.40 ± 0.42 in LAB only; (3) 31.20 ± 0.98 in bioactive fibers only; and (4) 51.10 ± 0.70 in placebo (nonfermentable fiber). The corresponding values of myeloperoxidase were (1) 25.62 ± 2.19, (2) 26.75 ± 2.61, (3) 56.59 ± 1.73 (3), and (4) $145.53 \pm$

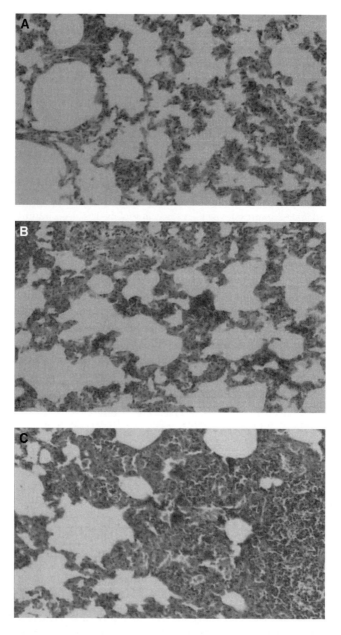

Fig. 1. Histologic sections of rat lungs 24 hours after cecal ligation and puncture (Mayer's hema-
toxylin, magnification × 100). (*A*) After placebo treatment. (*B*) After treatment with only bioactive
fibers. (*C*) After treatment with both bioactive fibers and live lactic acid bacteria (Synbiotic 2000).
(*Courtesy of* Dr. Ozer Ilkgul, Izmir, Turkey.)

7.53, respectively. Similarly, the changes in malone dialdehyde (MDA) were (1) 0.22 ± 1.31, (2) 0.28 ± 3.55, (3) 0.48 ± 5.32, and (4) 0.67 ± 2.94; and in nitric oxide, the values were (1) 17.16 ± 2.03, (2) 18.91 ± 2.24, (3) 47.71 ± 3.20, and (4) 66.22 ± 5.92. All differences between treatment groups and placebo were statistically significant ($P > .05$).

Prebiotics, probiotics, and synbiotics

Although the supplementation of LAB most often shows significant immunomodulatory effects in vitro and animal experiments, it sometimes fails when it comes to clinical trials. It is increasingly obvious that in LAB supplementation do only a minority of existing LAB that shows strong clinical immunomodulatory abilities. The experience from clinical studies is that the efficacy varies from none to significant as the treatment expands from single-strain to full flora replacement (treatment with donated feces by enemas): single-strain probiotic < multistrain probiotic or single-strain–single fiber synbiotics < multistrain–multifiber synbiotics < total fecal flora replacement [103,104].

Prebiotics

Prebiotics are substrates to be fermented by flora (eg, nondigestible food ingredients), mainly plant fibers, which will reach the colon undigested, food ingredients that are often referred to as colonic foods. Prebiotics are nutrients essential for the supply of substrate and energy for both flora and the host and that are essential for mucosal growth, water and electrolyte balance, and the body's resistance against invading pathogens. However, only one study has thus far tried only prebiotics in critically ill patients. Forty-one burn patients were randomized to receive either 6 g of oligofructose per day or sucrose as placebo during the first 15 days, but no difference in effect on lactulose/mannitol ratio or clinical outcome was observed between the groups [105].

Probiotics

Probiotics are live microorganisms from outside of the body supplied most commonly to the digestive tract. Most probiotics provided by dairy products or sold in health stores are not effective enough to be used in clinical medicine. Great differences exist in the ability of LAB to survive the passage through the GI tract and to influence cytokine production after passage through the stomach and small intestine, as demonstrated in a study in ileostomy patients [106]. Four different LAB species, *Lactobacillus plantarum*, *Lactobacillus paracasei*, *Lactobacillus rhamnosus*, and *Bifidobacter animalis*, were compared. Of the 10^8 cells/mL LAB originally administered orally of each LAB, only between 10^7 (*L plantarum*) and 10^2 (*L rhamnosus*) cells remained after the passage through the stomach and small intestine. Most of the strains tested after passage through the small intestine showed a significantly reduced or weak (especially *L rhamnosus*) ability to influence cytokine production (ie, the state of inflammation). Also, the ability to ferment fiber depends largely on the strain used, especially when applied on semiresistant prebiotics such as oligofructans inulin and phleins. When the oligofructans fermenting ability of 712 different LABs was studied, only 16 of 712 were able to ferment the phleins, and 8 of 712 were able to ferment inulin-type fiber [107]. Only four LAB species were able to ferment these fibers: *L plantarum* (several strains), *L paracasei* subsp *paracasei*, *L brevis,* and *Pediococcus pentosaceus.* The ability to control various pathogens is also strain-specific and limited to a few strains. When the ability of 50 different LABs to control 23 different pathogenic *Clostridium difficile* was tested, only 5 strains proved effective against all; 8 were antagonistic to some; but 27 were totally ineffective [108]. The five most effective strains were *L paracasei* subsp *paracasei* (two strains) and *L plantarum* (three strains).

Bovine milk not ideal as carrier of probiotics and synbiotics

It is important to recognize that cow's milk is not an ideal carrier of probiotics, especially when aimed for clinical use. In addition to its proposed role as a risk factor for increased inflammation in the body and development of ChDs [109], bovine milk does not, in contrast to breast milk, contain any fibers or fiber-like molecules (only elephant milk contains as much as human milk). Complex fucosylated oligosaccharides characteristic of human milk, with structural similarities to immunomodulating cell surface glycoconjugates (which enforce GI immunity and stimulate growth of health-supporting gut microflora), do not exist in bovine milk [110]. Cow's milk is not ideal as a carrier of probiotics and synbiotics because

1. It releases inflammatory mediators, induces inflammation, and induces leakage of molecules such as albumin and hyaluronan, increases intestinal permeability and causes translocation/leaky gut [111–116]
2. It is rich in AGE products produced during the heating-pasteurization process [117], particularly in milk powder, a common ingredient in clinical nutrition formulas (there is a direct association between the dietary intake of AGEs and the level of markers of systemic inflammation) [118]
3. It is rich in free polyunsaturated fats (shown also in lower concentrations than those in fermented dairy products to reduce the ability of LAB to adhere to mucous membranes and to grow) [119]
4. The colonization rate (ability to adhere to the mucosa and replicate) of so-called yoghurt bacteria is low (eg, *L casei* 2%; *L reuteri* 2%; and *L acidophilus* 0%) [120]
5. The LAB that can grow on milk substrates seem to lack clinical efficacy, as demonstrated in two recent controlled studies in postoperative and critically ill patients [121,122]

The lack of efficacy shown was shown in two studies that consisted of a standard commercial product (TREVIS, Ch Hansen, Denmark) containing *L acidophilus* LA5, *B lactis* BP12, *Streptococcus thermophilus*, and *L bulgaricus* mixed with 7.5 g of oligofructose, which was supplied to 45 critically ill ICU patients and 45 controls [121] and 72 elective abdominal surgery patients and 65 controls, respectively [122], in each study. The study of ICU patients reported a significant reduction in the number of PPMs in the stomach of the treated patients but no influence on intestinal permeability or any clinical benefits. The perioperative study reported no differences in bacterial translocation, gastric colonization, systemic inflammation, or septic complications [123].

Specific synbiotics for critically ill

A formula specifically intended for use in critically ill patients was developed in collaboration with Lund University microbiologists Åsa Ljungh and Torkel Wadström (produced commercially as Synbiotic 2000, Medipharm, Kågeröd, Sweden, and Des Moines, Iowa). The choice of LAB for the formulation was based on extensive studies of more than 350 human subjects [124] and over 180 plant microbial strains [125], which were selected especially for their abilities to produce bioactive proteins, transcribe NF-κB, produce proinflammatory and anti-inflammatory cytokines, produce antioxidants, and most important, to functionally complement each other. The formulation consists of a mixture of four bioactive LAB, one from each of the four main genera of Lactobacillus; 10^{10} *Pediococcus pentosaceus* 5-33:3, 10^{10} *Leuconostoc mesenteroides* 32-77:1, 10^{10} *L paracasei* subsp *paracasei* 19, and 10^{10} *L plantarum* 2362, that is, 40 billion LAB per dose, to which is added a mixture of four well-studied bioactive plant fibers: 2.5 g of betaglucan, 2.5 g of inulin, 2.5 g of pectin, and 2.5 g of resistant starch, for a total of 10 g of plant fibers. One or two such doses per day are administered to patients. In recent studies, a Synbiotic 2000 Forte and a Probiotic 2000 Forte (no fiber added) containing 10^{11} of each of the four LAB (ie, 400 billion LAB per dose were tried at the same dosing schedule of once or twice per day.

Multistrain-multifiber synbiotics in surgical and ICU patients

The synbiotic formulation has been tried in conditions such as acute pancreatitis, polytrauma, abdominal surgery, and chronic liver disease and liver transplantation.

Acute pancreatitis

Sixty-two patients who had severe acute pancreatitis (SAP) with acute physiology and chronic health evaluation (APACHE) II scores of synbiotic treated

11.7 ± 1.9 and controls 10.4 ± 1.5 were supplemented for 14 days with either two sachets per day of Synbiotic 2000 (2 × 40 billion LAB/d and 20 g total fiber) or with only the same amount of fiber (20 g) as in Synbiotic 2000. Nine of thirty-three patients (27%) in the Synbiotic 2000-treated group and 15 of 29 patients (52%) in the fiber only treated group developed subsequent infections. Eight of thirty-three (24%) Synbiotic 2000-treated patients, and 14 of 29 (48%) of the fiber only treated patients developed SIRS or MOF or both ($P < .005$) (A. Olah, personal communication, December 2005).

Polytrauma

Two studies using Synbiotic 2000 and Synbiotic 2000 Forte in polytrauma patients have been concluded, but the results are not yet published. One prospective randomized study conducted in patients who had acute extensive trauma compared supplementation with Synbiotic 2000 (40 billion LAB/d), a soluble fiber, a peptide diet, and glutamine. Treatment with Synbiotic 2000 led to a highly significant decrease in the number of chest infections (4/26 patients, 15%) compared with the peptide (11/26 patients, 42%; $P < .04$), glutamine (11/32 patients, 34%; $P < .03$), and fiber only diet (12/29 patients, 41%; $P < .002$). The total number of infections were also significantly decreased; Synbiotic 2000 (5/26 patients, 19%), fiber only (17/29 patients, 59%), peptide (13/26 patients, 50%), and glutamine diet (16/32 patients, 50%) (A. Spindler-Vesel, personal communication, 2005). In another study, 65 polytrauma patients were randomized to receive Synbiotic 2000 Forte or maltodextrin (placebo) once daily for 15 days. Significant reductions were observed in a number of parameters, such as the number of deaths (5/35 versus 9/30, respectively; $P < .02$), severe sepsis (6/35 versus 13/30, respectively; $P < .02$), chest infections (19/35 versus 24/30, respectively; $P < .03$), central line infections (13/32 versus 20/30, respectively; $P < .02$), and ventilation days (average 15 versus 26 days) (K. Kotzampassi, personal communication, 2005).

Abdominal surgery

In a controlled study, 45 patients undergoing major surgery for abdominal cancer were randomized to three treatment groups: enteral nutrition (EN) supplemented with Synbiotic 2000 (LEN); EN supplemented with only the fiber in the same amount (20 g) as in Synbiotic 2000 (FEN); and standard parenteral nutrition (PN). All treatments were initiated 2 days before surgery and continued to postoperative day 7. The incidence of postoperative bacterial infections was 47% with PN, 20% with FEN, and 6.7% with LEN ($P < .05$). Significant improvements were also observed in pre-albumin (LEN and FEN), C-reactive protein (LEN and FEN), serum cholesterol (LEN and FEN), white blood cell count (LEN), serum endotoxin (LEN and FEN), and IgA (LEN) [126].

Chronic liver disease and liver transplantation

Fifty-eight patients who had liver cirrhosis and so-called minimal encephalopathy were randomized into three treatment groups: group 1 (20 patients) received Synbiotic 2000; group 2 (20 patients) received the same amount of the fibers in Synbiotic 2000; and group 3 (15 patients) received placebo (nonfermentable, nonabsorbable crystalline cellulose fiber) [127]. A significant increase in intestinal LAB flora was observed after 1 month of supplementation in the Synbiotic-treated group 1 but not in the two other groups. Intestinal pH level was significantly reduced in both treatment groups 1 and 2 but not in the placebo-treated group 3. Significant decreases were observed in fecal counts of *Escherichia coli* and *Staphylococcus* and *Fusobacterium* but not in *Pseudomonas* and *Enterococcus*, and significant decreases in the levels of ammonia, endotoxins, alanine transaminase, and bilirubin (original level 252 ± 182) were observed in the synbiotic-treated group 1 (84 ± 65, $P < 0.01$) and in the fiber only treated group 2 (110 ± 86, $P < .05$), whereas levels remained unchanged in the placebo group 3. Equally important, the improvements in liver function were accompanied by significant improvements in psychometric tests and in the degree of encephalopathy. Later studies by the same group of investigators also showed significant improvements in liver blood flow and indocyanine clearance in patients supplemented for 1 week with Synbiotic 2000 [128]. These results offer great hope that synbiotic treatment given to patients awaiting liver transplantation could significantly reduce the number of septic episodes, improve liver function, and promote an improved outcome. Sixty-six patients were randomized to receive either Synbiotic 2000 or fiber only (same amount as in Synbiotic 2000) in connection with human orthotopic liver transplantation. The treatment started already on the day before surgery and continued for 14 days after surgery. During the first postoperative month, only one patient in the Synbiotic 2000-treated group (3%) showed signs of infection (urinary infection) compared with 17 of 33 (51%) patients in the group supplemented with only the four fibers [129]. The infecting organisms in the Synbiotic-treated group were *E faecalis* (1 patient); the organisms in the fiber only treated group were *E faecalis* and *E faecium* (11 patients), *E coli* (3 patients), *E cloacae* (2 patients), *P aeruginosa* (2 patients), and *Staph aureus* (1 patient). The use of antibiotics was on average 0.1 ± 0.1 days in the synbiotic-treated patients and 3.8 ± 0.9 days in the fiber-only treated group.

Immediate treatment is most important

The inflammatory response is immediate, and all attempts to control the response must therefore be immediate. Recent studies have demonstrated that immediate postoperative feeding using the enteral route is safe and prevents the increase in gut mucosal permeability. The enteral route is also reported to contribute to a positive nitrogen balance, to reduce the incidence of septic complications and the occurrence of postoperative ileus, and to accelerate restitution of pulmonary performance, body composition, and physical performance. An important observation is that delaying the supply of enteral nutrition for more than 24 hours results in a significant increase in intestinal permeability and a significantly higher incidence of MOF [130]. Oral or enteral nutrients supplied uninterruptedly during the night before, during surgery, and immediately thereafter seems to support the immune system and increase resistance to complications.

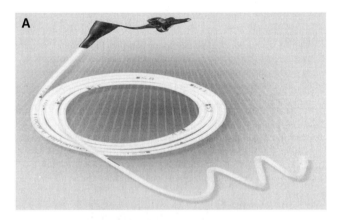

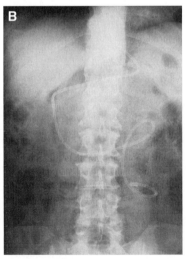

Fig. 2. (*A*) Bengmark auto-positioning regurgitation-resistant feeding tube. (*Courtesy of* Numico BV, Amsterdam, The Netherlands; with permission.) (*B*) Radiograph of a patient with the tube inserted. (*C*) Three-dimensional extraction CT scan of a patient with the tube in situ. (*D*) Intraoperative view showing the expansion of the tube in the small intestine. (*C–D*, *courtesy of* Dr. Gerardo Mangiante, Verona, Italy.)

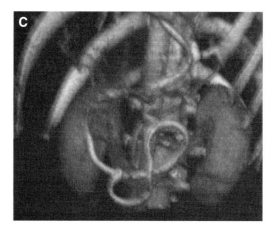

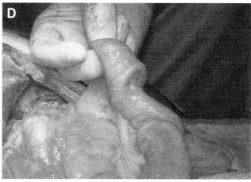

Fig. 2 (*continued*).

Regarding the day-to-day care of enteral nutrition, proper placement of a feeding tube, especially in critically ill patients who have impaired GI motility, can be a challenging task. The present author therefore developed an auto-positioning and regurgitation-resistant tube to facilitate the administration of enteral nutrition to eligible patients (Fig. 2). An early study has reported successful insertion, including in patients who have impaired GI motility, such as in SAP, and the head of the tube was reported to reach its optimal position in the upper small intestine in 10 of 10 patients within an average of 5.2 hours, and always within 24 hours [131]. Another more recent study reports the successful insertion in 12 of 16 (75%) acute pancreatitis patients, in whom the head of the tube reportedly reached the ligament of Treitz within a median of 12 hours [132]. An even more extensive study has reported successful placement within 24 hours of the tube placement in 78% of patients who had normal gastric emptying compared with 14% who had standard straight tubes ($P = .041$) and in 57% of patients who had impaired gastric emptying (eg, SAP patients) compared with 0% who had standard tubes ($P = .07$) [133].

Future aspects

Clearly, the ability of synbiotic treatment to modulate the acute phase response and reduce over-inflammation, as demonstrated particularly in animal
experiments, constitutes the most specific and significant effect of synbiotic
treatment in perioperative and critical care. A crucial condition for efficacy
and success in treatment is that the treatment is instituted before or at least
during the first few hours after trauma, which is possible in most emergency
medicine and surgery patients, such as in polytrauma. In some conditions, such
as severe acute pancreatitis, patients may arrive late in the hospital, which
clearly often reduces the efficacy of immunomodulatory and synbiotic treatment. Most patients in intensive care have already passed the acute nervous
phase and are in the deep immunoparalysis stage. Although no studies using
synbiotics in a general population of critical illness have yet concluded, it
seems most likely that less dramatic changes in clinical outcome will be the
result of such treatment. However, several controlled clinical studies are ongoing in a general population of ICU patients, the results of which are awaited
with the greatest interest.

Outcomes in critical illness seem to be dependent on numerous external,
internal, physical, mental, and environmental factors, which are known to have a
strong influence on genetic expression, particularly those associated with
inflammation. It is recommended that strong attempts are made to provide the
patients with a calm and silent environment and especially with sufficient sleep.
Disturbed rest and sleep are clearly associated with elevated levels of the
inflammatory markers such as IL-6 and sICAM [134]. Promoting vagal and Th1
functions through moderate feeding, hydration, and sleep, unexplained but
widely accepted recommendations for flu patients, is most likely also beneficial
in the treatment of critically ill patients.

Immunotoxicology and immunopharmacology are still in their infancy. Much
evidence exists to show that the drugs we use in ICUs largely have strong and
hitherto unrecognized influences on the immune system and the sensitivity to
inflammation and infection [135,136]. It is urgent that such influences are studied
and documented. It is a great dilemma that the sickest and most demanding
patients receive the most incomplete nutrition. There is an urgent need for new
enteral formulas. The formulas presently used are often adapted from parenteral
nutrition formulas and are intended to provide calories and to support a favorable
nitrogen balance. New insight necessitates formulas that are made mainly with
the goal to restore homeostasis in inflammation and immune functions. The new
science of nutrigenomics provides tools to identify the effects of various food
ingredients and their effects on various genes, particularly those associated with
inflammation and immune functions. Attempts can be made immediately to avoid
nutrition formula ingredients rich in saturated fat, *trans*-fatty acids, advanced
glycation products, hormones, and various stress molecules and sugars,
particularly fructose. Most important, the content of all such ingredients must
be carefully declared for each product.

Future enteral nutrition formulas will most likely be made to mimic normal food much more than is the case today. There is a need to undertake studies to compare the effects of normal foods versus hospital-made enteral nutrition formulas with commercial standard clinical nutrition formulas on outcome, especially in critically ill patients. Certainly, regular foods, such as Mediterranean soups like gazpacho and various other vegetable and fish soups, can be adapted for clinical use and, at least to begin with, used as a complement to commercial enteral nutrition formulas. Fresh fruit and vegetable juices should frequently be used in the ICUs. Fruit and vegetable mixers are important therapeutic tools in the ICU. LAB, fibers, and antioxidants (not only or mainly vitamins), various polyphenols such as curcumenoids and resveratrol and similar molecules, and plant- and animal-based foods should be considered.

Recent information demonstrates that critically ill patients suffer not only an overgrowth of pathogens in the GI tract but have lost their entire beneficial LAB flora [137], which is information that might provide support for supplementing lactic acid bacteria and restoring homeostasis in flora to ICU patients. Recent cutting-edge study results from the supplementation of synbiotics to post-operative and critically ill patients support the recommendation of routinely supplying specific LAB and fibers (synbiotics) both to patients who have acute pancreatitis and polytrauma as well as to those undergoing extensive medical or surgical treatments. For patients who cannot tolerate enteral feeding, the administration of synbiotics by enemas or, in the future, by subcutaneous injections (vaccination) with live LAB may be treatment options. Most important, enteral nutrition aimed at preventing hyperinflammation and subsequent complications should be instituted as early as possible, even as a priority in the emergency room.

References

[1] Arias E, Smith BL. Deaths: preliminary data for 2001. Natl Vital Stat Rep 2003;51:1–44.
[2] Angus DC, Linde-Zwirble WT, Lidicker J, et al. Epidemiology of severe sepsis in the United States: analysis of incidence, outcome and associated costs of care. Crit Care Med 2001;29: 1303–10.
[3] Vincent J-L, Abraham E, Annane D, et al. Reducing mortality in sepsis: new directions. Crit Care 2002;6(Suppl 3):S1–18.
[4] Angus DC, Wax RS. Epidemiology of sepsis: an update. Crit Care Med 2001;29:109–16.
[5] van Nieuwenhoven CA, Buskens E, van Tiel FH, et al. Relationship between methodological trial quality and the effects of selective digestive decontamination on pneumonia and mortality in critically ill patients. JAMA 2001;286:335–40.
[6] Isenmann R, Runzi M, Kron M, et al. Prophylactic antibiotic treatment in patients with pre-dicted severe acute pancreatitis: a placebo-controlled, double-blind trial. Gastroenterology 2004;126:997–1004.
[7] Dellinger EP, Tellado JM, Soto N and Study 89 Investigator Group. Prophylactic antibiotic treatment in patients with severe acute necrotizing pancreatitis: a double blind placebo-controlled study. Presentation K-1374, Abstract to 45th ICAAC, American Society for Microbiology 2005.

 [8] Kox WJ, Volk T, Kox SN, et al. Immunomodulatory therapies in sepsis. Intensive Care Med 2000;26(Suppl 1):S124–8.

 [9] Feldmann M, Brennan FM, Paleolog E, et al. Anti-TNFalpha therapy of rheumatoid arthritis: what can we learn about chronic disease? Novartis Found Symp 2004;256:53–69.

[10] World Health Organization. Process for a global strategy on diet, physical activity and health. Geneva (Switzerland): World Health Organization; 2003.

[11] Bengmark S. Acute and "chronic" phase response–a mother of disease. Clin Nutr 2004;23:1256–66.

[12] Bengmark S. Bio-ecological control of the gastrointestinal tract: the role of flora and sup-plemented pro- and synbiotics. Gastroenterol Clin North Am 2005;34:413–36.

[13] Bengmark S. Impact of nutrition on ageing and disease. Curr Opin Nutr Metab Care 2006;9: 2–7.

[14] Schwartz MN. Hospital-acquired infections; diseases with increasingly limited therapies. Proc Natl Acad Sci U S A 1994;91:2420–6.

[15] Bengmark S. Nutritional modulation of acute and "chronic" phase response. Nutrition 2001; 17:489–95.

[16] Costa M, Brookes SJ, Hennig GW. Anatomy and physiology of the enteric nervous system. Gut 2000;47(Suppl 4):S15–9.

[17] Lyte M. Microbial endocrinology and infectious disease in the 21st century. Trends Microbiol 2004;12:14–20.

[18] Groves AC, Griffiths J, Leung F, et al. Plasma catecholamines in patients with serious postoperative infection. Ann Surg 1973;178:102–7.

[19] Kinney KS, Austin CE, Morton DS, et al. Norepinephrine as a growth stimulating factor in bacteria: mechanistic studies. Life Sci 2000;67:3075–85.

[20] Alverdy JC, Laughlin RS, Wu L. Influence of the critically ill state on host-pathogen inter-actions within the intestine: gut-derived sepsis redefined. Crit Care Med 2003;31:598–607.

[21] Halonen KI, Leppäniemi AK, Lundin JE, et al. Prediction fatal outcome in the early phase of severe acute pancreatitis by using novel prognostic models. Pancreatology 2003;3:309–15.

[22] Imrie CW. Prognostic indicators in acute pancreatitis. Can J Gastroenterol 2003;17:325–8.

[23] Roszkowski K, Ko KL, Beuth J, et al. Intestinal microflora of BALB/c-mice and function of local immune cells. Zentralbl Bacteriol Mikrobiol Hyg (A) 1988;270:270–9.

[24] Calabrese EJ, Baldwin LA. Hormesis as a biological hypothesis. Environ Health Perspect 1998;106(Suppl 1):S357–62.

[25] Lange H. Multiorgan dysfunction syndrome: how water might contribute to its progression. J Cell Mol Med 2002;6:653–60.

[26] Lobo DN, Bostock KA, Neal KR, et al. Effect of salt and water balance on recovery of gastrointestinal function after elective colonic resection: a randomised controlled trial. Lancet 2002;359:1812–8.

[27] Macafee DAL, Allison SP, Lobo DN. Some interactions between gastrointestinal function and fluid and electrolyte homeostasis. Curr Opin Clin Nutr Metab Care 2005;8:197–203.

[28] Wan JMF, Teo TC, Babayan VK, et al. Lipids and the development of immune dysfunction. JPEN J Parenter Enteral Nutr 1988;12(Suppl 6):S43–52.

[29] Van der Poll T, Coyle SM, Levi M, et al. Fat emulsion infusion potentiates coagulation activation during human endotoxemia. Thromb Haemost 1996;75:83–6.

[30] Lin BF, Huang CC, Chiang BL, et al. Dietary fat influences Ia antigen expression, cytokines and prostaglandin E_2 production in immune cells in autoimmune-prone NZBxNZW F1 mice. Br J Nutr 1996;75:711–22.

[31] Umpierrez GE, Isaacs SD, Bazargan N, et al. Hyperglycemia: an independent marker of in-hospital mortality in patients with undiagnosed diabetes. J Clin Endocrinol Metab 2002;87: 978–82.

[32] Mesotten D, Van den Berghe G. Clinical potential of insulin therapy in critically ill patients. Drugs 2003;63:625–36.

[33] Lind L, Lithell H. Impaired glucose and lipid metabolism seen in intensive care patients is related to severity of illness and survival. Clin Intensive Care 1994;5:100–5.

[34] Klein CJ, Stanek GS, Wiles CE. Overfeeding macronutrients to critically ill adults: metabolic complications. J Am Diet Assoc 1998;98:795–806.

[35] Sandström R, Drott C, Hyltander A, et al. The effect of postoperative intravenous feeding (TPN) on outcome following major surgery evaluated in a randomized study. Ann Surg 1993; 217:185–95.

[36] Heslin MJ, Latkany L, Leung D, et al. A prospective randomized trial of early enteral feeding after resection of upper gastrointestinal malignancy. Ann Surg 1997;226:567–80.

[37] Biffl WL, Moore EE, Moore FA, et al. Interleukin-6 delays neutrophil apoptosis via a mechanism involving platelet-activating factor. J Trauma 1996;40:575–9.

[38] Alessi MC, Peiretti F, Morange P, et al. Production of plasminogen activator inhibitor 1 by human adipose tissue: possible link between visceral fat accumulation and vascular disease. Diabetes 1997;46:860–7.

[39] Thomas EL, Saeed N, Hajnal JV, et al. Magnetic resonance imaging of total body fat. J Appl Physiol 1998;85:1778–85.

[40] Menges T, Engel J, Welters I, et al. Changes in blood lymphocyte populations after multiple trauma. Crit Care Med 1999;27:733–40.

[41] Zahorec R. Ratio of neutrophil to lymphocyte counts–rapid and simple parameter of systemic inflammation and stress in critically ill. Bratisl Lek Listy 2001;102:5–14.

[42] Kalff C, Carlos TM, Schraut WH, et al. Surgically induced leukocytic infiltrates within the rat intestinal muscularis mediate postoperative ileus. Gastroenterology 1999;117:378–87.

[43] De Jonge WJ, Van den Wungaard RM, The FO, et al. Postoperative ileus is maintained by intestinal immune infiltrates that activate inhibitory neural pathways in mice. Gastroenterology 2003;125:1137–47.

[44] Steinberg KP, Milberg JA, Martin TA, et al. Evolution of bronchoalveolar cell populations in the adult respiratory distress syndrome. Am J Respir Crit Care Med 1994;150:113–22.

[45] Sookhai S, Wang JH, McCourt M, et al. A novel mechanism for attenuating neutrophil-mediated lung injury in vivo [abstract]. Surg Forum 1999;50:205–8.

[46] Wei L, Wei H, Frenkel K. Sensitivity to tumor promotion of SENCAR and C57BL/6J mice correlates with oxidative events and DNA damage. Carcinogenesis 1993;14:841–7.

[47] Kubes P, Hunter J, Granger DN. Ischemia/reperfusion induced feline intestinal dysfunction: importance of granulocyte recruitment. Gastroenterology 1992;103:807–12.

[48] Ho JS, Buchweitz JP, Roth RA, et al. Identification of factors from rat neutrophil responsible for cytotoxicity to isolated hepatocytes. J Leukoc Biol 1996;59:716–24.

[49] Lowell CA, Bertin G. Resistance to endotoxic shock and reduced neutrophil migration in mice deficient for the Src-family kinases Hck and Fgr. Proc Natl Acad Sci U S A 1998;95:7580–4.

[50] Goris BJA, te Boekhorst TPA, Nuytinck JKS, et al. Multiple-organ failure: generalized autodestructive inflammation. Arch Surg 1985;120:1109–15.

[51] Wilson MR, Choudhury S, Takata M. Pulmonary inflammation induced by high-stretch ventilation is mediated by tumor necrosis factor signalling in mice. Am J Physiol Lung Cell Mol Physiol 2005;288:L599–607.

[52] Rassias AJ, Marrin CAS, Arruda J, et al. Insulin infusion improves neutrophil function in diabetic cardiac surgery patients. Anaesth Analg 1999;88:1011–6.

[53] ÓBrien G, Shields CJ, Winter DC, et al. Cyclooxygenase-2 plays a central role in the genesis of pancreatitis and associated lung injury. Hepatobiliary Pancreat Dis Int 2005;4:126–9.

[54] Bengmark S. Curcumin: an atoxic antioxidant and natural NF-κB, COX-2, LOX and iNOS inhibitor: a shield against acute and chronic diseases. JPEN J Parenter Enteral Nutr 2006; 30:45–51.

[55] Taneja R, Parodo J, Jia SH, et al. Delayed neutrophil apoptosis in sepsis is associated with maintenance of mitochondrial transmembrane potential and reduced caspase-9 activity. Crit Care Med 2004;32:1460–9.

[56] Johnson CD, Abu-Hilal M for the British Acute Pancreatitis Study Group. Persistent organ failure during the first week as a marker of fatal outcome in acute pancreatitis. Gut 2004; 53:1340–4.

[57] McKay CJ, Buter A. Natural history of organ failure in acute pancreatitis. Pancreatoloy 2003;3: 111-4.

[58] Gómez-Cambronera LG, Sabater L, Pereda J, et al. Role of cytokines and oxidative stress in the pathophysiology of acute pancreatitis: therapeutic implications. Curr Drug Targets Inflamm Allergy 2002;1:393-403.

[59] Gonzales RJ, Moore EE, Ciesla DJ, et al. Post-hemorrhagic shock mesenteric lymph activates human pulmonary microvascular endothelium for in vitro neutrophil-mediated injury–the role of intracellular adhesion molecule-1. J Trauma 2003;54:219-23.

[60] Deitch EA, Shni HP, Feketeova E, et al. Serine proteases are involved in the pathogenesis of trauma-hemorrhagic shock-induced gut and lung injury. Shock 2003;19:452-6.

[61] Deitch EA, Shi HP, Skurnick J, et al. Mesenteric lymph from burned rats induces endothelial cell injury and activates neutrophils. Crit Care Med 2004;32:533-8.

[62] Goodman RB, Pugin J, Lee JS, et al. Cytokine-mediated inflammation in acute lung injury. Cytokine Growth Factor Rev 2003;14:523-35.

[63] Deitch EA, Forsythe R, Anjaria D, et al. The role of lymph factors in lung injury, bone marrow suppression, and endothelial cell dysfunction in a primate model of trauma-hemorrhagic shock. Shock 2004;22:221-8.

[64] Aller MA, Arias JL, Arias J. Post-traumatic inflammatory response: perhaps a succession of phases with a nutritional purpose. Med Hypotheses 2004;63:42-6.

[65] Kerlin BA, Yan B, Isenmann BH, et al. Survival advantage associated with heterozygous factor V Leiden mutation in patients with severe sepsis and in mouse endotoxemia. Blood 2003;102: 3085-92.

[66] Texereau J, Pene F, Chiche JD, et al. Importance of hemostatic gene polymorphisms for susceptibility to and outcome of severe sepsis. Crit Care Med 2004;32(Suppl 5):S313-9.

[67] Bengmark S. Bio-ecological control of acute pancreatitis; the role of enteral nutrition, pro- and synbiotics. Curr Opin Nutr Metab Care 2005;8:557-61.

[68] Sautner T, Fugger R, Götzinger P, et al. Tumour necrosis factor-α and interleukin-6: early indicators of bacterial infection after human orthotopic liver transplantation. Eur J Surg 1995; 161:97-101.

[69] Estenssoro E, Gonzáles F, Laffaire E, et al. Shock on admission day is the best predictor of prolonged mechanical ventilation in the ICU. Chest 2005;127:598-603.

[70] Bochicchio GV, Salzano L, Joshi M, et al. Admission preoperative glucose is predictive of mortality and morbidity in trauma patients who require immediate operative intervention. Am Surg 2005;71:171-4.

[71] Bochicchio GV, Sung J, Joshi M, et al. Persistent hyperglycemia is predictive of outcome in critically ill trauma patients. J Trauma 2005;58:921-4.

[72] Muehlstedt SC, Lyte M, Rodriguez JL. Increased IL-10 production and HLA-DR suppression in lungs of injured patients precede the development of nosocomial pneumonia. Shock 2002; 17:443-50.

[73] Pachot A, Monneret G, Brion A, et al. Messenger RNA expression of major histocompatibility complex class II genes in whole blood from septic shock patients. Crit Care Med 2005;33: 31-8.

[74] Mentula P, Kylanpaa-Back ML, Kemppainen E, et al. Decreased HLA (human leukocyte antigen)-DR expression on peripheral blood monocytes predicts the development of organ failure in patients with acute pancreatitis. Clin Sci (Lond) 2003;105:409-17.

[75] Mentula P, Kylenpää M-L, Kemppainen E, et al. Plasma anti-inflammatory cytokines and monocyte human leukocyte antigen-DR expression in acute pancreatitis. Scand J Gastroenterol 2004;39:178-87.

[76] Yu W-K, Li W-Q, Li N, et al. Mononuclear histocompatibility leukocyte antigen-DR expression in the early phase of acute pancreatitis. Pancreatology 2004;4:233-43.

[77] Oczenski W, Krenn H, Jilch R, et al. HLA-DR as a marker for increased risk of systemic inflammation and septic complications after cardiac surgery. Intensive Care Med 2003;29: 1253-7.

[78] Hidemura A, Saito H, Fukatsu K, et al. Patients with postoperative infections have sticky neutrophils before operation. Shock 2003;19:497–502.

[79] Bengmark S. Bioecological control of perioperative and ITU morbidity. Langenbecks Arch Surg 2004;389:145–54.

[80] Bengmark S. Bioecological control of inflammation and infection in transplantation. Transplant Rev 2004;18:38–53.

[81] Engelich G, Wright DG, Hartshorn KL. Acquired disorders of phagocyte function complicating medical and surgical illnesses. Clin Infect Dis 2001;33:2040–8.

[82] Laird AM, Miller PR, Kilgo PD, et al. Relationship of early hyperglycemia to mortality in trauma patients. J Trauma 2004;56:1058–62.

[83] Deitch EA, Shorshtein A, Houghton J, et al. Inducible nitric oxide synthase knockout mice are resistant to diet-induced loss of gut barrier function and intestinal injury. J Gastrointest Surg 2002;6:599–605.

[84] Hill GE, Frawley WH, Griffith KE, et al. Allogeneic blood transfusion increases the risk of postoperative bacterial infection: a metaanalysis. J Trauma 2003;54:908–14.

[85] Mayer K, Fegbeutel C, Hattar K, et al. ω-3 vs ω-6 lipid emulsions exert differential influence on neutrophils in septic shock patients: impact on plasma fatty acids and lipid mediator generation. Int Care Med 2003;29:1472–81.

[86] Nathens AB, Neff MJ, Jurkovich GJ, et al. Randomized, prospective trial of antioxidant supplementation in critically ill surgical patients. Ann Surg 2002;236:814–22.

[87] Baines M, Shenkin A. Use of antioxidants in surgery: a measure to reduce postoperative complications. Curr Opin Clin Nutr Metab Care 2002;5:665–70.

[88] Bengmark S. Use of pro-, pre- and synbiotics in the ICU–future options. In: Shikora SA, Martindale RG, Schwaitzberg SD, editors. Nutritional considerations in the intensive care unit – science, rationale and practice. Dubuque (IA): Kendall/Hunt Publishing; 2002. p. 381–99.

[89] Bengmark S. Aggressive peri- and intraoperative enteral nutrition–strategy for the future. In: Shikora SA, Martindale RG, Schwaitzberg SD, editors. Nutritional considerations in the intensive care unit–science, rationale and practice. Dubuque (IA): Kendall/Hunt Publishing; 2002. p. 365–80.

[90] Bengmark S. Synbiotics and the mucosal barrier in critically ill patients. Curr Opin Gastroenterol 2005;21:712–6.

[91] Heyman M. Effect of lactic acid bacteria on diarrheal diseases. J Am Coll Nutr 2000; 19(Suppl 2):S137–46.

[92] Husebye E, Hellstrom PM, Sundler F, et al. Influence of microbial species on small intestinal myoelectric activity and transit in germ-free rats. Am J Physiol Gastrointest Liver Physiol 2001; 280:G368–80.

[93] Verdu EF, Bercik P, Bergonzelli GE, et al. Lactobacillus paracasei normalizes muscle hypercontractility in a murine model of postinfective gut dysfunction. Gastroenterology 2004; 127(3):826–37.

[94] Kelly D, Campbell JI, King TP, et al. Commensal anaerobic gut bacteria attenuate inflammation by regulating nuclear-cytoplasmic shuttling of PPAR-gamma and RelA. Nat Immunol 2004; 5:104–12.

[95] Bai AP, Ouyang Q, Zhang W, et al. Probiotic inhibit TNF-α-induced interleukin-8 secretion of HT29 cells. World J Gastroenterol 2004;10:455–7.

[96] Petrof EO, Kojima K, Ropeleski MJ, et al. Probiotics inhibit nuclear factor-kappaB and induce heat shock proteins in colonic epithelial cells through proteasome inhibition. Gastroenterology 2004;127:1474–87.

[97] Ma D, Forsythe P, Bienenstock J. Live Lactobacillus reuteri is essential for inhibitory effect on tumor necrosis factor alpha-induced interleukin-8 expression. Infect Immun 2004;72: 5308–14.

[98] Nurmi JT, Puolakkainen PA, Rautonon NE. Bifidobacterium lactis sp 420 up-regulates cyclooxygenase (Cox)-1 and downregulates Cox-2 gene expression in a Caco-2 cell culture model. Nutr Cancer 2005;5:83–92.

[99] Fink MP. Ethyl pyruvate: a novel treatment for sepsis and shock. Minerva Anestesiol 2004;
      70:365–71.

[100] Oxman T, Shapira M, Diver A, et al. A new method of long-term preventive cardioprotection
      using *Lactobacillus*. Am J Physiol Heart Circ Physiol 2000;278:H1717-24.

[101] Ilkgul O, Bengmark S, Aydede H, et al. Pretreatment with pro- and synbiotics reduces
      peritonitis-induce lung injury in rats. In press.

[102] Ilkgul O, Aydede H, Erhan Y, Surucuoglu S, et al. Subcutaneous administration of live
      lactobacillus prevents sepsis-induced lung organ failure in rats. Br J Int Care 2005;15:52–7.

[103] Borodo TJ, Warren EF, Leis S, et al. Treatment of ulcerative colitis using fecal bacteriotherapy.
      J Clin Gastroenterol 2003;37:42–7.

[104] Borody TJ, Warren EF, Leis SM, et al. Bacteriotherapy using fecal flora: toying with human
      motions. J Clin Gastroenterol 2004;38:475–83.

[105] Olguin F, Araya M, Hirsch S, et al. Prebiotic ingestion does not improve gastrointestinal barrier
      function in burn patients. Burns 2005;31:482–8.

[106] Miettinen M, Alander M, von Wright A, et al. The survival of and cytokine induction by lactic
      acid bacteria after passage through a gastrointestinal model. Microb Ecol Health Dis 1998;10:
      41–147.

[107] Müller M, Lier D. Fermentation of fructans by epiphytic lactic acid bacteria. J Appl Bacteriol
      1994;76:406–11.

[108] Naaber P, Smidt I, Stsepetova J, et al. Inhibition of *Clostridium difficile* strains by intestinal
      Lactobacillus species. J Med Microbiol 2004;53:551–4.

[109] Solomons NW. Nature's perfect food revisited: recent insights on milk consumption and
      chronic disease risk. Nutr Rev 2002;60:180–2.

[110] Gnoth MJ, Kunz C, Kinne-Saffran E, et al. Human milk oligosaccharides are minimally
      digested in vitro. J Nutr 2000;130:3014–20.

[111] Kalliomaki M, Salminen S, Arvilommi H, et al. Probiotics in primary prevention of atopic
      disease: a randomized placebo-controlled trial. Lancet 2001;357:1076–9.

[112] Jalonen T. Identical intestinal permeability changes in children with different clinical
      manifestations of cow's milk allergy. J Allergy Clin Immunol 1991;88:737–42.

[113] Isolauri E, Majamaa H, Arvola T, et al. *Lactobacillus casei* strain GG reverses increased intes-
      tinal permeability induced by cow milk in suckling rats. Gastroenterology 1993;105:1643–50.

[114] Bengtsson U, Knutson TW, Knutson L, et al. Increased levels of hyaluronan and albumin after
      intestinal challenge in adult patients with cow's milk intolerance. Clin Exp Allergy 1996;26:
      96–103.

[115] Bengtsson U, Knutson TW, Knutson L, et al. Eosinophil cationic protein and histamine after
      intestinal challenge in patients with cow's milk intolerance. J Allergy Clin Immunol 1997;100:
      216–21.

[116] Ehn BM, Ekstrand B, Bengtsson U, et al. Modification of IgE binding during heat processing of
      the cow's milk allergen. J Agric Food Chem 2004;52:1398–403.

[117] Ahmed N, Mirshekar-Syahkal B, Kennish L, et al. Assay of advanced glycation end products in
      selected beverages and food by liquid chromatography with tandem mass spectrometric
      detection. Mol Nutr Food Res 2005;49:691–9.

[118] Uribarri J, Cai W, Sandu O, et al. Diet-derived advanced glycation end products are major
      contributors to the body's AGE pool and induce inflammation in healthy subjects. Ann N Y
      Acad Sci 2005;1043:461–6.

[119] Kankanpää PE, Salminen SJ, Isolauri E, et al. The influence of polyunsaturated fatty acids on
      probiotic growth and adhesion. FEMS Microbiol Lett 2001;194:149–53.

[120] Ahrné S, Nobaek S, Jeppsson B, et al. The normal *Lactobacillus* flora of healthy human rectal
      and oral mucosa. J Appl Microbiol 1998;85:88–94.

[121] Jain PK, McNaught CE, Anderson ADG, MacFie J, et al. Influence of synbiotic containing
      Lactobacillus acidophilus LA5, *Bifidobacterium lactis* BP12, *Streptococcus thermophilus*,
      Lactobacillus bulgaricus and oligofructose on gut barrier function and sepsis in critically ill
      patients: a randomized controlled trial. Clin Nutr 2004;23:467–75.

[122] Woodcock NP, McNaught CE, Morgan DR, et al. An investigation into the effect of a probiotic on gut immune function in surgical patients. Clin Nutr 2004;23:1069–73.

[123] Bengmark S. Synbiotics to strengthen gut barrier function and reduce morbidity in critically ill patients. Clin Nutr 2004;23:441–5.

[124] Ljungh Å, Lan JG, Yamagisawa N. Isolation, selection and characteristics of *Lactobacillus paracasei* ssp *paracasei* isolate F19. Microb Ecol Health Dis 2002;14(Suppl 3):4–6.

[125] Kruszewska K, Lan J, Lorca G, et al. Selection of lactic acid bacteria as probiotic strains by in vitro tests. Microecology and Therapy 2002;29:37–51.

[126] Han Chunmao, Martindale R, Huang H, et al. Pre- and postoperative enteral supply of a synbiotic composition reduces the incidence of postoperative septic complications in abdominal cancer surgery. In press.

[127] Liu Q, Duan ZP, Ha DK, et al. Synbiotic modulation of gut flora: effect on minimal hepatic encephalopathy in patients with liver cirrhosis. Hepatology 2004;39:1441–9.

[128] Kurtovic J, Ruettimann U, Adamson H, et al. Improvement in indocyanine green clearance following synbiotic treatment in cirrhosis [abstract]. Gut 2003;52:A3.

[129] Rayes N, Seehofer D, Theruvath T, et al. Combined perioperative enteral supply of bioactive pre- and probiotics abolishes postoperative bacterial infections in human liver transplantation: a randomized, double blind clinical trial. Am J Transplant 2005;5:125–30.

[130] Kompan L, Kremzar B, Gadzijev E, et al. Effects of early enteral nutrition on intestinal permeability and the development of multiple organ failure after multiple injury. Intensive Care Med 1999;25:129–30.

[131] Mangiante G, Colucci G, Marinello P, et al. Bengmark's selfpropelling naso-jejunal tube: a new useful device for intensive enteral nutrition [abstract]. Intensive Care Med 1998;24:330.

[132] Karsenti D, Viguiler J, Bourlier P, et al. Enteral nutrition during acute pancreatitis: feasibility study of a self-propelling spiral distal end jejunal tube. Gastroenterol Clin Biol 2003;27:614–7.

[133] Lai CWY, Barlow R, Barnes M, et al. Bedside placement of nasojejunal tubes: a randomized-controlled trial of spiral vs straight-ended tubes. Clin Nutr 2003;22:267–70.

[134] Motivala SJ, Sarfatti A, Olmos L, et al. Inflammatory markers and sleep disturbance in major depression. Psychosom Med 2005;67:187–94.

[135] Hadden JW. Immunopharmacology and immunotoxicology. Adv Exp Med Biol 1991;288:1–11.

[136] Descotes J. Immunotoxicology: role in the safety assessment of drugs. Drug Saf 2005;28:127–36.

[137] Knight DJW, Ala'Aldeen D, Bengmark S, et al. The effect of synbiotics on gastrointestinal flora in the critically ill. Br J Anaesth 2004;92:307–8.

ELSEVIER
SAUNDERS

Anesthesiology Clin N Am
24 (2006) 325–340

ANESTHESIOLOGY
CLINICS OF
NORTH AMERICA

Linking Stress to Inflammation

Angelika Bierhaus*, Per M. Humpert, Peter P. Nawroth

Department of Medicine I, INF 410, University of Heidelberg, Heidelberg 69120, Germany

The stress system orchestrates body and brain responses to the environment, thus sensing for danger and at the same time aiming to maintain homeostasis. This response ensures the survival of organisms in situations in which they face exogenous and endogenous stressors. Under conditions of acute aggression, the body elicits a "flight or fight" reaction by activating a set of rather stereotyped neuroendocrine and inflammatory responses, with certain similarities between infection, trauma, or psychosocial stress situations. The defense reaction of the body involves not only the activation of the sympathetic nervous system and the hyopothalamic-pituary-adrenal (HPA) axis but also proinflammatory transcription factors, cytokines, coagulation factors, and vasoconstrictors. Thus, the response to psychosocial stress bears a close but as yet poorly understood relationship with inflammation. This article summarizes the current knowledge of the overlap of stress, inflammation, and immune response.

Transcription factors: central mediators in the cellular response to psychosocial stress

Both major and minor stressful events can have direct adverse effects on a variety of inflammatory and immunologic mechanisms. In vitro studies and studies in animals and humans imply that these immune alterations may be detrimental, with serious consequences to health [1]. One molecular link between psychosocial stress and organ function is provided by the activation of the proinflammatory transcription factor nuclear factor κB (NF-κB). NF-κB controls

This work was supported by a grant from the Manfred-Lautenschläger-Stiftung for the Study of Diabetes (PPN).
* Corresponding author.
E-mail address: angelika_bierhaus@med.uni-heidelberg.de (A. Bierhaus).

doi:10.1016/j.atc.2006.01.001

the expression of the majority of genes required for the cellular defense and also regulates the activity of cytokine-producing immune cells [2,3]. Bound to inhibitory molecules of the IκB family in the cytoplasm, NF-κB is rapidly activated by a variety of inflammatory and metabolic signals (Fig. 1). On activation, NF-κB translocates into the nucleus and activates genes required to ensure survival [4].Therefore, NF-κB activation is recognized as the central mediator of inflammatory and immune responses in life-threatening situations such as septicemia [5], Crohn's disease and colitis [6,7], arteriosclerosis, coronary heart disease [8], and diabetes mellitus [2,4,7,9–15]. In all these settings, blockage of excessive NF-κB activation has been shown to relate to a better outcome of the disease. Recent studies have extended our understanding of

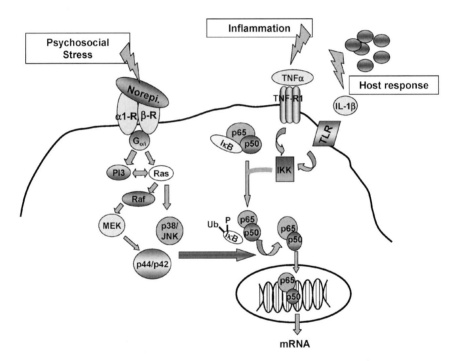

Fig. 1. Proposed signaling mechanism of psychosocial stress and cytokine-dependent cellular activation Stress-induced norepinephrine (Norepi.) binds to α1- and β-adrenergic receptors (R), causing G-protein-dependant activation of Ras, Raf, and MAP kinases, which induces as yet uncharacterized signaling pathways, resulting in the phosphorylation and degradation of the NF-κB-specific cytoplasmic inhibitor IκBα and subsequent activation and nuclear translocation of NF-κB [123]. Cytokines activate NF-κB through a variety of receptors, such as TNF receptors or Toll-like receptors (TLR) and downstream interaction with NIK induces the formation of large IKK complexes, which in turn phosphorylate IκBα and trigger nuclear translocation of NF-κB [124]. The unifying intracellular signal of stress and inflammatory cytokines is the activation of NF-κB-dependent proinflammatory, proadhesive, and procoagulant gene expression. IKK, IκB kinase; JNK, c-Jun N-terminal kinase; MAPK, mitogen-activated protein kinases; MEK, mitogen-activated protein kinase/extracellular signal-regulated kinase kinase; NIK, NF-κB-inducing kinase.

NF-κB as a central molecule in response to a danger by showing that acute mental stress is sufficient to induce NF-κB nuclear translocation in peripheral blood mononuclear cells (pBMC) (see Fig. 1) [16]. The activation of NF-κB in pBMC of healthy volunteers subjected to the Trier Social Stress Test (TSST), which consists of performing a short free speech and an arithmetic test in front of an audience [17], was observed in most of the volunteers within 10 minutes (Fig. 2) [16]. Remarkably, the degree of NF-κB-activation in pBMC correlated with the stress-dependent increase in catecholamines and cortisol levels [16]. When the stressful situation had resolved, NF-κB activation rapidly returned to basal levels within 60 minutes, in the majority of the responsive participants [16], whereas some volunteers were unable to down-regulate NF-κB within this time frame [16]. The latter implies an individual stress perception and stress management, which may contribute by the personal risk for stress-related disease [18–23].

A similar activation of NF-κB activation and NF-κB-dependent gene expression was observed in animal experiments in which mice were exposed to a mild restraint stress [16]. Stress-related NF-κB activation and subsequent gene expression are most likely mediated by norepinephrine-induced (and not epinephrine) α_1/β-adrenoreceptor-dependent signaling cascades [16]. Physiologically, norepinephrine is released from sympathetic nerve fibers in direct approximation to target tissues and thus provides the organism with the hormone to initiate a response to an immediate threat [24]. Remarkably, noradrenergic sympathetic nerve fibers not only regulate vascular and muscle tone but, in addition, connect the central nervous system (CNS) with primary and secondary lymphoid organs [25], implying a direct modulation of immune cells in the

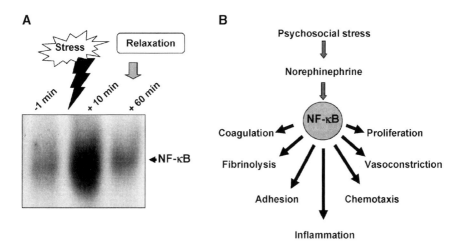

Fig. 2. Psychosocial stress-dependent NF-κB activation in the pBMC of healthy volunteers. (A) Course of NF-κB binding activity in pBMC during a short laboratory stress test monitored by electrophoretic mobility shift assay [16,17]. (B) Proposed consequences of stress-induced NF-κB activation and subsequent NF-κB-dependent gene expression.

acute stress response [24]. Because both physiologic concentrations of norepi-nephrine in vitro and a short activation of the sympathoadrenergic axis in vivo are sufficient to induce an NF-κB-triggered proinflammatory cellular response, repeated episodes or chronic exposure to catecholamines may be sufficient to induce dysfunctional inflammatory and immune reactions. Furthermore, NF-κB activation disrupts glucocorticoid receptor signaling and promotes glucocorticoid resistance, thereby altering glucocorticoid-mediated feedback reactions [26].

In addition to NF-κB activation, catecholamine binding to adrenergic re-ceptors results in activation of the cAMP response element binding protein (CREB), which also induces the transcription of cytokines. β-adrenergic-induced G-protein activation results in the activation of adenylate cyclase, which in turn catalyzes the synthesis of cAMP from ATP [27,28]. The cAMP-dependent protein kinase A phosphorylates CREB, which subsequently induces CREB-regulated genes such as interleukin (IL)-6.

The inflammatory reflex: cytokines link the central nervous and immune systems

The bidirectional communication between the immune system and the brain is mediated mostly by proinflammatory cytokines [29,30]. Inflammatory processes are signaled to the brain by macrophages using cytokines such as tumor necrosis factor (TNF)-α, IL-1, and IL-6. In response, the CNS reacts by sending out autonomic reflexes mediated by norepinephrine and is capable of modulating immune processes. Therefore, cytokines are regarded as principal mediators between the CNS and the immune system, ensuring adequate reactions to inflammatory diseases [29–31].

Consistent with the close connection between psychosocial stress and NF-κB activation and the innate immune response and inflammation, a number of studies provide compelling evidence that psychosocial stress primarily stimulates the production of proinflammatory cytokines. Increased plasma concentrations of IL-1β, IL-2, and IL-6 were detected in volunteers undergoing acute laboratory stress tests [32,33] as well as in individuals expecting an academic examination [34]. In particular, IL-6 reactivity was identified as an independent predictor of stress-induced cellular changes [35].

Acute stressors directly induce the expression of IL-1β in inflammatory cells [36,37]. IL-1β expression is dependent on NF-κB [38] and in turn activates IL-6 [39,40]. In laboratory stress tests, healthy men demonstrated a significant increase in IL-1β gene expression 30 minutes after stress, which correlated positively with plasma IL-6-response, cardiovascular responses, subjective stress ratings, and anxiety symptoms [41]. In addition to IL-1β-dependent IL-6 activation, the increase in IL-6 is likely to be mediated by direct adrenergic effects, because physiologic concentrations of norepinephrine have been shown to increase IL-6 mRNA in cultured monocytic cells [16].

Murine models of social stress have furthermore demonstrated that social disruption results in the increased TNF-α secretion from both CD11b$^+$ monocytes and splenocytes, pointing to the complex interaction underlying the cellular response to psychosocial stress [42]. Experiments studying cytokine release on lipopolysaccharide stimulation after a laboratory speech test in healthy volunteers, however, demonstrated an increase in IL-6, whereas TNF-α production remained unchanged [43]. Moreover, the infusion of isoproterenol, a β-adrenergic agonist, blunted TNF-α-production, whereas IL-6 synthesis was unaffected [43]. In contrast, β-adrenergic stimulation increased the gene expression of TNF-α, IL-1β, and IL-6 in myocardial cells [44]. A norepinephrine-dependent α-adrenoreceptor-mediated increase in TNF-α has been reported in Kupffer cells [45], whereas α1- and β-receptors contribute to the norepinephrine-dependent IL-6 induction in THP-1 monocytic cells (see Fig. 1) [16].

Although IL-6 is commonly classified as a proinflammatory cytokine, it also exhibits inhibitory properties reflected by the up-regulation of IL-1-receptors and stimulation of the HPA axis [43,46]. The importance of IL-6 in mediating the cellular response to psychosocial stress was confirmed recently in IL-6$^{-/-}$ mice [47]. In experiments in which cage-switching stress was applied to male wild type (WT) or IL-6$^{-/-}$ mice, the cage switching increased the mean arterial pressure in the IL-6-bearing WT mice but was significantly blunted in IL-6-deficient mice [47]. In contrast, there were no differences in either an increase in heart rate and motor activity, plasma renin activity, or plasma norepinephrine concentrations [47]. Because IL-6$^{-/-}$ mice have elevated norepinephrine baseline levels, it cannot excluded that receptor desensitization or reduced responsiveness to sympathetic stimulation might have contributes to the attenuated hypertensive response [47]. Although the underlying molecular mechanism has still to be deciphered, these data clearly demonstrate that the acute hypertensive response to psychosocial stress significantly depends on IL-6. The diversity of results, however, implies a differential cell-specific and receptor-specific regulation of cytokines by the sympathetic nervous system.

Inflammatory reflex: immune cells as a primary target of sympathoadrenergic cell activation

Monocytes, macrophages, lymphocytes, and granulocytes bear receptors for both neuroendocrine products of the sympathetic adrenal-medullary (SAM) and the HPA axes [24]. Thus, the psychosocial stress-induced adrenergic activation of SAM and HPA can directly target transcription factor activation and change gene expression in immune cells. A recent clinical study with healthy physicians indicated that a short mental test is sufficient to up-regulate the plasma levels of NF-κB-controlled adhesion molecules such as intercellular adhesion molecule (ICAM)-1 [32]. Acute stress also increases the number of ICAM-1-expressing inflammatory monocytes, lymphocytes, and granulocytes [48–50]. In particular, the increase in Leukocyte function-associated antigen (LFA-1; CD11a/CD18) [50] and Mac-1-positive lymphocytes [51] correlated with the increase in catecholamine plasma levels. LFA-1 and Mac-1 are ligands of ICAM-1 [52]. Because ICAM-1 is expressed on both, leukocytes and endothelial cells, psychosocial stress might directly promote leukocyte adhesion to endothelial cells and endothelial dysfunction. CD11a and CD11b adhesion molecules have also been shown to be involved in stress-induced alterations in T-cell distribution further implying, that stress-hormone-dependent alterations of adhesion molecule expression on immune and endothelial cells may contribute to stress-induced changes in leukocyte activation. Social disruption in a murine model of social stress increases the number of CD11b$^+$ monocytes, but reduces their responsiveness to the inhibitory effects of glucocorticoids [42]. Furthermore, acute stress events increase the chemotactic response of pBMC to N-formyl-methyl-leucyl-phenylalanine (fMLP) and stromal-derived factor 1 (SDF-1) [51,53].

Consistently, social stress enhances leukocyte trafficking of all leukocyte subpopulations. Although chronic stress is immune suppressive [54], acute stress seems to increase leukocyte trafficking [54,55]. An acute laboratory stress test with 56 healthy volunteers has demonstrated a significant stress-dependent increase in cytotoxic T-cells natural killer cell activity (NKCA) that was paralleled by an increased interferon-γ release from pBMC [56]. A recently performed experiment in which surgical sponges were implanted in acutely stressed mice to determine the extent of leukocyte infiltration confirmed an increase of up to 300% in neutrophils, macrophages, natural killer (NK)-cells, and T-cell infiltration compared with nonstressed animals [55]. This finding is in line with previous studies showing enhanced cutaneous immune function during acute stress [57]. Therefore, it is supposed that acute stress may prepare immune cells to face challenges that might occur during the expected fight-or-flight reaction. Although stress-induced leukocyte trafficking is beneficial in promoting immune protection during wounding and infection, it will doubtless also exacerbate stress-induced inflammatory and autoimmune processes and thus potentially promote diseases such as cardiovascular disease, arthritis, or psoriasis [55].

Stress, inflammation, and coagulation: dysbalanced defense strategies?

The simultaneous activation of the immune response and the coagulation system represents an evolutionarily conserved system and an essential part of the host defense response, with the aim of restoring cellular integrity in situations in which the endothelial surface might be destroyed [58]. Consistently, healthy volunteers undergoing a short laboratory stress test have demonstrated a stress-dependent increase in the coagulation factors FVII, FVIII, and FXIII as well as in thrombin–antithrombin (TAT) complexes. The induction of TAT complexes positively correlated with β2-adrenergic sensitivity and the release of norepinephrine [59]. Both inflammation and norepinephrine-dependent activation of NF-κB result in the induction of tissue factor (TF), the major mediator of extrinsic coagulation. Factor VIII is also up-regulated by NF-κB [60]. Recent in vitro studies have demonstrated a dose- and time-dependent increase in TF mRNA synthesis in response to physiologic concentrations of norepinephrine (A. Bierhaus and colleagues, 2005). Experimental stress models in db/db mice also indicate that restraint stress is sufficient to induce TF expression and subsequent fibrin formation in smooth muscle and epithelial cells as well as in adipocytes [61]. Remarkably, this stress model, however, was not sufficient to induce TF synthesis in endothelial cells [61]. These observations imply the presence of as yet unidentified cell-specific protection mechanisms that may protect vascular cells from TF expression in situations of acute stress. Consistently, recent observations in healthy volunteers have demonstrated that a negative effect was associated with attenuated procoagulant reactivity to stress, whereas the opposite was observed for a positive effect [62]. In contrast, a similar short laboratory stress test performed in distressed dementia caregivers evoked an acute procoagulant stress response, suggesting that higher combined caregiving and life distress levels are associated with more dysfunctional hemostatic responses to acute mental stress [63]. Female teachers [64] also demonstrated increased fibrinogen-dimer and fibrin D-dimer levels, arguing for an increased prothrombotic activity in situations of chronic stress. One special feature of the stress-dependent activation of coagulation is the absence of habituation effects in response to repeated stress episodes [65]. This implies that the coagulation system is unable to adapt to stress and indicates a direct stress-dependent impairment of the vascular system and its hemostatic properties [65]. The coagulation–inflammation cycle in response to chronic stress exposure is further promoted by the fact that thrombin is able to activate NF-κB and to perpetuate the initial proinflammatory response [66]. Furthermore, coagulation promotes the inflammatory state by generating hemostatic proteinases [67] and protease-activated receptors that elicit inflammatory gene expression [68].

Plasminogen activator inhibitor-1 (PAI1) is another gene that is regulated partly by NF-κB, and norepinephrine-mediated NF-κB-activation potentially results in increased PAI1 and decreased fibrinolytic activity. Although a direct proof is missing, a variety of experimental and clinical studies indicates reduced fibrinolysis on stress exposure. In obese mice, acute stress results in a highly significant increase in PAI1 transcription, expression, and plasma levels [69]. A number of clinical studies further describe reduced fibrinolysis resulting from increased PAI1 and decreased tissue-plasminogen activator (tPA) plasma concentrations, particularly in subjects who have chronic stress burden, such as healthy volunteers with vital exhaustion [70–72] or high job stress [64,73] and patients with chronic back pain [74]. Furthermore, acute psychosocial stressors seem to be sufficient to reduce the tPA/PAI1 coefficient in patients who have cardiovascular diseases [75].

Hence, it seems likely that initially protective coagulation responses to acute psychosocial stress can be overrun, depending on the quality, duration, and individual perception of the stressor, leading finally to a procoagulant state and unfavorable modulation of inflammatory reflexes.

Inflammation-mediated vasoconstriction: linking stress to hypertension?

Psychosocial stress triggers an increase in endothelin (ET)-1 plasma levels in both healthy volunteers and patients who have cardiovascular disease [76]. To date, it is not clear if this increase is caused by the induction of new ET-1 synthesis or the increased release of preformed ET-1. ET-1 transcription, however, is regulated at least in part by NF-κB [77], and recent observations indicate that physiologic concentrations of norepinephrine induce preproendothelin mRNA in cultured endothelial cells (A. Bierhaus and colleagues, 2005). Furthermore, there is evidence that IL-6 is able to cause or facilitate vasoconstriction by increasing ET_B receptor-mediated contraction [78,79], thus implying that the activation of inflammatory mediators may contribute to the reported increase in ET-1 on a psychosocial challenge.

Inflammatory reflex: cholinergic activity counteracts sympathetic inflammatory response

Psychosocial stress-induced activation of inflammation has been interpreted as part of the body's survival-oriented sickness response. This implies the existence of mechanisms able to down-regulate the cellular response as soon as the challenge has been resolved. Recently, it was demonstrated that the efferent vagus nerve is able to blunt the proinflammatory cytokine release and thus to protect against inflammation playing a major role in neuroimmunomodulation [80–82]. It is generally believed that the vagal afferent nerve pathway dominates the response to mild to moderate peripheral inflammation, whereas strong inflammatory signals are transmitted to the brain through humoral mechanisms [83]. Whether the transmission of cytokine signals to the brain occurs through vagal sensory neurons, therefore, depends on the magnitude of the immune challenge. Vagal afferents can be activated either directly by cytokines released from dendritic cells and immune cells, particularly macrophages, or indirectly through chemoreceptive cells located in vagal paraganglia [83]. This results directly or indirectly through nucleus tractus solitarius neuron-mediated activation of vagal efferents in the dorsal motor nucleus of the vagus. Because vagal efferents are distributed throughout the periphery and the brain-derived motor output through the vagus efferent neurons is rapid, the vagus controls and modulates the peripheral inflammatory status [84–86]. In doing so, the cholinergic efferent fibers signal directly to macrophages and microvascular endothelial cells, which have been recently identified to express the α7 subunits of the nicotinic acetylcholine receptor and to exert cholinergic anti-inflammatory pathways [81,85,87,88]. The essential role of the α7-nicotinic acetylcholine receptor subunit in mediating the activity of cholinergic anti-inflammatory pathways has been demonstrated in α7-subunit$^{-/-}$ mice, in which vagal withdrawal promotes inflammation (Fig. 3) [81]. To date, however, data are missing that

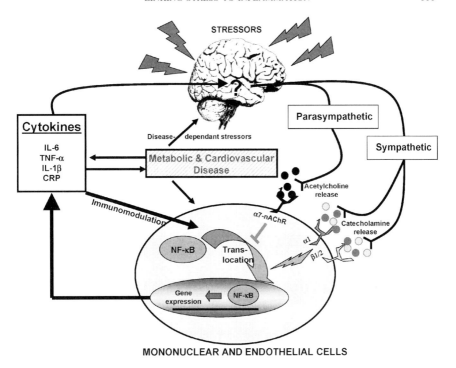

Fig. 3. The autonomic inflammatory reflex psychosocial stressors lead to activation of the sympathetic and parasympathetic autonomic nervous system, causing a release of catecholamines and acetylcholine from autonomic nerve endings. These neurotransmitters can bind to adrenergic ($\alpha 1/\beta 1/\beta 2$) and cholinergic receptors on endothelial and mononuclear cells, leading to distinct cellular changes. Although noradrenalin causes a translocation of NF-κB into the nucleus and subsequent expression of inflammatory genes [16], binding of acetylcholine to the $\alpha 7$ subunit of nicotinic acetylcholine receptor ($\alpha 7$-nAChR) leads to the inhibition of inflammatory cell activation [81]. Adrenergic activation of immune and endothelial cells leads to the expression and release of cytokines that have been shown to play a role in the development of metabolic and cardiovascular disease. Because inflammatory cytokines such as TNF-α, IL-1, and IL-6 signal inflammation to the CNS, an unbalanced and stress-dependant activation of the sympathetic system could cause a vicious cycle, aggravating inflammatory and metabolic disease. CRP, C-reactive protein.

show a direct involvement of cholinergic anti-inflammatory pathways in the resolution of psychosocial stress-induced inflammation.

Psychosocial stress, inflammation, and the pathway to metabolic disease

Most of the studies on the influence of psychosocial stress cited above have been conducted in healthy volunteers subjected to short-lasting mental stress in experimental settings. However, little is known about the consequences of chronic psychosocial stress that afflicts millions of people all over the world on cellular signaling and the expression of proinflammatory or procoagulant gene products [89]. There is, however, some evidence that inflammatory markers, such as C-reactive protein, IL-6 [90–92], as well as procoagulant factors [63,70,93,94] are elevated in subjects suffering from chronic stress. As discussed above, inflammatory and procoagulant states can be a consequence of sympathetic adrenal–medullary or hypothalamic–pituitary–adrenal activation during chronic psychosocial stress. Both pathways have been shown to cause insulin resistance [95–103], which can be considered as one central pathophysiologic mechanism in the development of the metabolic syndrome, diabetes, and cardiovascular disease. A possible link among chronic stress, insulin resistance, and the development of cardiovascular disease (and other inflammatory diseases) may be chronic or repeated activation of NF-κB, which has been shown recently to be activated by mental stress and β-adrenergic signaling [16]. In this case, the NF-κB-dependent expression of IL-6 and other inflammatory cytokines under chronic stress could directly influence insulin sensitivity [104], as shown recently in hepatocellular cells and adipocytes [92,105,106]. Consistently, increased levels of IL-6 have been reported in patients under chronic stress [95] as well as in patients who have metabolic and cardiovascular disease [107–109]. In patients already suffering from metabolic diseases, the unfavorable effects of stress-dependent NF-κB may become even more deleterious [110–113]. In consequence, the overexpression of inflammatory cytokines such as IL-6 could not only exaggerate the metabolic state but also signal to the CNS, as described above, evoking an autonomic reflex and causing a vicious cycle of systemic inflammation (see Fig. 3).

Summary

There is ample evidence for the influence of central nervous system modulation through inflammatory cellular reactions under psychosocial stress. These inflammatory reflexes might be of major influence not only for metabolic and vascular disease but also for many autoimmune diseases for which stress has been reported as a risk factor [114–116]. In prospective trials on the influence of risk factors for the occurrence of cardiovascular events, both psychosocial stress and autonomic nervous control of the cardiovascular system were shown to have a major impact on event rates [20,117–120]. The underlying cause of these findings seems to be explained in part by the direct influences of autonomic reflexes, potentially induced by psychosocial tasks, on the progression of atherosclerosis [121,122].

Hence, future prospective studies that aim at deciphering the influence of chronic psychosocial stress and autonomic function on the pathogenesis of inflammatory and metabolic disease will need to include neurophysiologic, molecular, and clinical parameters. Because the neuroimmunologic axis can be seen as a system connecting mental states with inflammatory reactions, pro-inflammatory mediators and anti-inflammatory strategies should be studied as such in experimental settings.

References

[1] Tappy L, Seematter G, Martin JL. Environmental influences on diseases in later life. Nestle Nutr Workshop Ser Clin Perform Programme 2004;19–30 [discussion: 30–15].
[2] Mercurio F, Manning AM. NF-kappaB as a primary regulator of the stress response. Oncogene 1999;18:6163–71.
[3] Xiao C, Ghosh S. NF-kappaB, an evolutionarily conserved mediator of immune and inflammatory responses. Adv Exp Med Biol 2005;560:41–5.
[4] Barnes PJ, Karin M. Nuclear factor-kappaB: a pivotal transcription factor in chronic inflammatory diseases. N Engl J Med 1997;336:1066–71.
[5] Bohrer H, Qiu F, Zimmermann T, et al. Role of NFkappaB in the mortality of sepsis. J Clin Invest 1997;100:972–85.
[6] Neurath MF, Pettersson S. Predominant role of NF-kappa B p65 in the pathogenesis of chronic intestinal inflammation. Immunobiology 1997;198:91–8.
[7] Thiele K, Bierhaus A, Autschbach F, et al. Cell specific effects of glucocorticoid treatment on the NF-kappaBp65/IkappaBalpha system in patients with Crohn's disease. Gut 1999;45:693–704.
[8] Valen G, Yan ZQ, Hansson GK. Nuclear factor kappa-B and the heart. J Am Coll Cardiol 2001;38:307–14.
[9] Hofmann MA, Schiekofer S, Isermann B, et al. Peripheral blood mononuclear cells isolated from patients with diabetic nephropathy show increased activation of the oxidative-stress sensitive transcription factor NF-kappaB. Diabetologia 1999;42:222–32.
[10] Hofmann MA, Schiekofer S, Kanitz M, et al. Insufficient glycemic control increases nuclear factor-kappa B binding activity in peripheral blood mononuclear cells isolated from patients with type 1 diabetes. Diabetes Care 1998;21:1310–6.
[11] Evans JL, Goldfine ID, Maddux BA, et al. Oxidative stress and stress-activated signaling pathways: a unifying hypothesis of type 2 diabetes. Endocr Rev 2002;23:599–622.
[12] Mohamed AK, Bierhaus A, Schiekofer S, et al. The role of oxidative stress and NF-kappaB activation in late diabetic complications. Biofactors 1999;10:157–67.
[13] Mattson MP, Camandola S. NF-kappaB in neuronal plasticity and neurodegenerative disorders. J Clin Invest 2001;107:247–54.
[14] Bierhaus A, Nawroth PP. Modulation of the vascular endothelium during infection–the role of NF-kappa B activation. Contrib Microbiol 2003;10:86–105.
[15] Bierhaus A, Haslbeck KM, Humpert PM, et al. Loss of pain perception in diabetes is dependent on a receptor of the immunoglobulin superfamily. J Clin Invest 2004;114:1741–51.
[16] Bierhaus A, Wolf J, Andrassy M, et al. A mechanism converting psychosocial stress into mononuclear cell activation. Proc Natl Acad Sci U S A 2003;100:1920–5.
[17] Kirschbaum C, Pirke KM, Hellhammer DH. The 'Trier Social Stress Test'–a tool for investigating psychobiological stress responses in a laboratory setting. Neuropsychobiology 1993;28:76–81.
[18] Kawakami N, Takatsuka N, Shimizu H, et al. Depressive symptoms and occurrence of type 2 diabetes among Japanese men. Diabetes Care 1999;22:1071–6.
[19] Nakata A, Haratani T, Takahashi M, et al. Job stress, social support, and prevalence of insomnia in a population of Japanese daytime workers. Soc Sci Med 2004;59:1719–30.
[20] Rosengren A, Hawken S, Ounpuu S, et al. Association of psychosocial risk factors with risk of acute myocardial infarction in 11119 cases and 13648 controls from 52 countries (the INTERHEART study): case-control study. Lancet 2004;364:953–62.
[21] Keltikangas-Jarvinen L, Kettunen J, Ravaja N, et al. Inhibited and disinhibited temperament and autonomic stress reactivity. Int J Psychophysiol 1999;33:185–96.
[22] Kawakami N, Araki S, Takatsuka N, et al. Overtime, psychosocial working conditions, and occurrence of non-insulin dependent diabetes mellitus in Japanese men. J Epidemiol Community Health 1999;53:359–63.
[23] Keltikangas-Jarvinen L, Ravaja N, Viikari J. Identifying Cloninger's temperament profiles as

related to the early development of the metabolic cardiovascular syndrome in young men. Arterioscler Thromb Vasc Biol 1999;19:1998–2006.

[24] Padgett DA, Glaser R. How stress influences the immune response. Trends Immunol 2003;24: 444–8.

[25] Felten SY, Felten DL, Bellinger DL, et al. Noradrenergic and peptidergic innervation of lymphoid organs. Chem Immunol 1992;52:25–48.

[26] Raison CL, Miller AH. When not enough is too much: the role of insufficient glucocorticoid signaling in the pathophysiology of stress-related disorders. Am J Psychiatry 2003;160: 1554–65.

[27] Vallejo M. Transcriptional control of gene expression by cAMP-response element binding proteins. J Neuroendocrinol 1994;6:587–96.

[28] Todd PK, Mack KJ. Phosphorylation, CREB, and mental retardation. Pediatr Res 2001;50:672.

[29] Johnson JD, Campisi J, Sharkey CM, et al. Catecholamines mediate stress-induced increases in peripheral and central inflammatory cytokines. Neuroscience 2005;135:1295–307.

[30] Elenkov IJ, Iezzoni DG, Daly A, et al. Cytokine dysregulation, inflammation and well-being. Neuroimmunomodulation 2005;12:255–69.

[31] Hosoi T, Okuma Y, Nomura Y. The mechanisms of immune-to-brain communication in inflammation as a drug target. Curr Drug Targets Inflamm Allergy 2002;1:257–62.

[32] Heinz A, Hermann D, Smolka MN, et al. Effects of acute psychological stress on adhesion molecules, interleukins and sex hormones: implications for coronary heart disease. Psychopharmacology (Berl) 2003;165:111–7.

[33] Steptoe A, Willemsen G, Owen N, et al. Acute mental stress elicits delayed increases in circulating inflammatory cytokine levels. Clin Sci (Lond) 2001;101:185–92.

[34] Maes M, Van Der Planken M, Van Gastel A, et al. Influence of academic examination stress on hematological measurements in subjectively healthy volunteers. Psychiatry Res 1998;80: 201–12.

[35] von Kanel R, Kudielka BM, Hanebuth D, et al. Different contribution of interleukin-6 and cortisol activity to total plasma fibrin concentration and to acute mental stress-induced fibrin formation. Clin Sci (Lond) 2005;109:61–7.

[36] Brydon L, Edwards S, Mohamed-Ali V, et al. Socioeconomic status and stress-induced increases in interleukin-6. Brain Behav Immun 2004;18:281–90.

[37] Brydon L, Steptoe A. Stress-induced increases in interleukin-6 and fibrinogen predict ambulatory blood pressure at 3-year follow-up. J Hypertens 2005;23:1001–7.

[38] Hiscott J, Marois J, Garoufalis J, et al. Characterization of a functional NF-kappa B site in the human interleukin 1 beta promoter: evidence for a positive autoregulatory loop. Mol Cell Biol 1993;13:6231–40.

[39] Frangogiannis NG, Smith CW, Entman ML. The inflammatory response in myocardial infarction. Cardiovasc Res 2002;53:31–47.

[40] Fraser JK, Lill MC, Figlin RA. The biology of the cytokine sequence cascade. Semin Oncol 1996;23:2–8.

[41] Brydon L, Edwards S, Jia H, et al. Psychological stress activates interleukin-1beta gene expression in human mononuclear cells. Brain Behav Immun 2005;19:540–6.

[42] Avitsur R, Kavelaars A, Heijnen C, et al. Social stress and the regulation of tumor necrosis factor-alpha secretion. Brain Behav Immun 2005;19:311–7.

[43] Goebel MU, Mills PJ, Irwin MR, et al. Interleukin-6 and tumor necrosis factor-alpha production after acute psychological stress, exercise, and infused isoproterenol: differential effects and pathways. Psychosom Med 2000;62:591–8.

[44] Murray DR, Prabhu SD, Chandrasekar B. Chronic beta-adrenergic stimulation induces myocardial proinflammatory cytokine expression. Circulation 2000;101:2338–41.

[45] Zhou M, Yang S, Koo DJ, Ornan DA, et al. The role of Kupffer cell alpha(2)-adrenoceptors in norepinephrine-induced TNF-alpha production. Biochim Biophys Acta 2001;1537:49–57.

[46] Papanicolaou DA, Wilder RL, Manolagas SC, et al. The pathophysiologic roles of interleukin-6 in human disease. Ann Intern Med 1998;128:127–37.

[47] Lee DL, Leite R, Fleming C, et al. Hypertensive response to acute stress is attenuated in interleukin-6 knockout mice. Hypertension 2004;44:259–63.

[48] Goebel MU, Mills PJ. Acute psychological stress and exercise and changes in peripheral leukocyte adhesion molecule expression and density. Psychosom Med 2000;62:664–70.

[49] Mills PJ, Dimsdale JE. The effects of acute psychologic stress on cellular adhesion molecules. J Psychosom Res 1996;41:49–53.

[50] Mills PJ, Farag NH, Hong S, et al. Immune cell CD62L and CD11a expression in response to a psychological stressor in human hypertension. Brain Behav Immun 2003;17:260–7.

[51] Redwine L, Snow S, Mills P, Irwin M. Acute psychological stress: effects on chemotaxis and cellular adhesion molecule expression. Psychosom Med 2003;65:598–603.

[52] McEver RP. Adhesive interactions of leukocytes, platelets, and the vessel wall during hemostasis and inflammation. Thromb Haemost 2001;86:746–56.

[53] Redwine L, Mills PJ, Sada M, et al. Differential immune cell chemotaxis responses to acute psychological stress in Alzheimer caregivers compared to non-caregiver controls. Psychosom Med 2004;66:770–5.

[54] Dhabhar FS, McEwen BS. Acute stress enhances while chronic stress suppresses cell-mediated immunity in vivo: a potential role for leukocyte trafficking. Brain Behav Immun 1997;11:286–306.

[55] Viswanathan K, Dhabhar FS. Stress-induced enhancement of leukocyte trafficking into sites of surgery or immune activation. Proc Natl Acad Sci U S A 2005;102:5808–13.

[56] Larson MR, Ader R, Moynihan JA. Heart rate, neuroendocrine, and immunological reactivity in response to an acute laboratory stressor. Psychosom Med 2001;63:493–501.

[57] Dhabhar FS. Stress, leukocyte trafficking, and the augmentation of skin immune function. Ann N Y Acad Sci 2003;992:205–17.

[58] Bierhaus A, Nawroth PP. [Coagulation, inflammation and immune response–an evolutionary conserved plan as cause for disseminated intravasal coagulation?] Hamostaseologie 2005;25:23–32 [in German].

[59] von Kanel R, Mills PJ, Ziegler MG, et al. Effect of beta2-adrenergic receptor functioning and increased norepinephrine on the hypercoagulable state with mental stress. Am Heart J 2002;144:68–72.

[60] Begbie M, Notley C, Tinlin S, et al. The factor VIII acute phase response requires the participation of NFkappaB and C/EBP. Thromb Haemost 2000;84:216–22.

[61] Yamamoto K, Shimokawa T, Yi H, et al. Aging and obesity augment the stress-induced expression of tissue factor gene in the mouse. Blood 2002;100:4011–8.

[62] von Kanel R, Kudielka BM, Preckel D, et al. Opposite effect of negative and positive affect on stress procoagulant reactivity. Physiol Behav 2005;86:61–8.

[63] von Kanel R, Dimsdale JE, Patterson TL, et al. Acute procoagulant stress response as a dynamic measure of allostatic load in Alzheimer caregivers. Ann Behav Med 2003;26:42–8.

[64] Fenga C, Micali E, Cacciola A, et al. Stressful life events and fibrinogen level in middle-aged teachers. Psychopathology 2004;37:64–8.

[65] von Kanel R, Preckel D, Zgraggen L, et al. The effect of natural habituation on coagulation responses to acute mental stress and recovery in men. Thromb Haemost 2004;92:1327–35.

[66] Minami T, Abid MR, Zhang J, et al. Thrombin stimulation of vascular adhesion molecule-1 in endothelial cells is mediated by protein kinase C (PKC)-delta-NF-kappa B and PKC-zeta-GATA signaling pathways. J Biol Chem 2003;278:6976–84.

[67] Strukova S. Blood coagulation-dependent inflammation: coagulation-dependent inflammation and inflammation-dependent thrombosis. Front Biosci 2006;11:59–80.

[68] Chu AJ. Tissue factor mediates inflammation. Arch Biochem Biophys 2005;440:123–32.

[69] Strike PC, Magid K, Brydon L, et al. Exaggerated platelet and hemodynamic reactivity to mental stress in men with coronary artery disease. Psychosom Med 2004;66:492–500.

[70] Vrijkotte TG, van Doornen LJ, de Geus EJ. Work stress and metabolic and hemostatic risk factors. Psychosom Med 1999;61:796–805.

[71] Kop WJ, Hamulyak K, Pernot C, et al. Relationship of blood coagulation and fibrinolysis to vital exhaustion. Psychosom Med 1998;60:352–8.

[72] von Kanel R, Frey K, Fischer J. Independent relation of vital exhaustion and inflammation to fibrinolysis in apparently healthy subjects. Scand Cardiovasc J 2004;38:28–32.

[73] Ishizaki M, Tsuritani I, Noborisaka Y, et al. Relationship between job stress and plasma fibrinolytic activity in male Japanese workers. Int Arch Occup Environ Health 1996;68:315–20.

[74] Graver V, Haaland AK, Loeb M, et al. Fibrinolytical activity in relation to psychological traits in patients with sciatica. Thromb Res 1997;85:363–6.

[75] Hevey D, McGee HM, Fitzgerald D, et al. Acute psychological stress decreases plasma tissue plasminogen activator (tPA) and tissue plasminogen activator/plasminogen activator inhibitor-1 (tPA/PAI-1) complexes in cardiac patients. Eur J Appl Physiol 2000;83:344–8.

[76] Mangiafico RA, Malatino LS, Attina T, et al. Exaggerated endothelin release in response to acute mental stress in patients with intermittent claudication. Angiology 2002;53:383–90.

[77] Quehenberger P, Bierhaus A, Fasching P, et al. Endothelin 1 transcription is controlled by nuclear factor-kappaB in AGE-stimulated cultured endothelial cells. Diabetes 2000;49:1561–70.

[78] Leseth KH, Adner M, Berg HK, et al. Cytokines increase endothelin ETB receptor contractile activity in rat cerebral artery. Neuroreport 1999;10:2355–9.

[79] White LR, Juul R, Skaanes KO, et al. Cytokine enhancement of endothelin ET(B) receptor-mediated contraction in human temporal artery. Eur J Pharmacol 2000;406:117–22.

[80] Borovikova LV, Ivanova S, Zhang M, et al. Vagus nerve stimulation attenuates the systemic inflammatory response to endotoxin. Nature 2000;405:458–62.

[81] Wang H, Yu M, Ochani M, Amella CA, et al. Nicotinic acetylcholine receptor alpha7 subunit is an essential regulator of inflammation. Nature 2003;421:384–8.

[82] Metz CN, Tracey KJ. It takes nerve to dampen inflammation. Nat Immunol 2005;6:756–7.

[83] Pavlov VA, Tracey KJ. The cholinergic anti-inflammatory pathway. Brain Behav Immun 2005;19:493–9.

[84] Andersson J. The inflammatory reflex–introduction. J Intern Med 2005;257:122–5.

[85] Czura CJ, Tracey KJ. Autonomic neural regulation of immunity. J Intern Med 2005;257:156–66.

[86] Tracey KJ. The inflammatory reflex. Nature 2002;420:853–9.

[87] Saeed RW, Varma S, Peng-Nemeroff T, et al. Cholinergic stimulation blocks endothelial cell activation and leukocyte recruitment during inflammation. J Exp Med 2005;201:1113–23.

[88] de Jonge WJ, van der Zanden EP, The FO, et al. Stimulation of the vagus nerve attenuates macrophage activation by activating the Jak2-STAT3 signaling pathway. Nat Immunol 2005;6:844–51.

[89] Korte SM, Koolhaas JM, Wingfield JC, et al. The Darwinian concept of stress: benefits of allostasis and costs of allostatic load and the trade-offs in health and disease. Neurosci Biobehav Rev 2005;29:3–38.

[90] Melamed S, Shirom A, Toker S, et al. Association of fear of terror with low-grade inflammation among apparently healthy employed adults. Psychosom Med 2004;66:484–91.

[91] Jeanmonod P, von Kanel R, Maly FE, et al. Elevated plasma C-reactive protein in chronically distressed subjects who carry the A allele of the TNF-alpha-308 G/A polymorphism. Psychosom Med 2004;66:501–6.

[92] Kiecolt-Glaser JK, Preacher KJ, MacCallum RC, et al. Chronic stress and age-related increases in the proinflammatory cytokine IL-6. Proc Natl Acad Sci U S A 2003;100:9090–5.

[93] von Kanel R, Dimsdale JE, Patterson TL, et al. Association of negative life event stress with coagulation activity in elderly Alzheimer caregivers. Psychosom Med 2003;65:145–50.

[94] Raikkonen K, Lassila R, Keltikangas-Jarvinen L, et al. Association of chronic stress with plasminogen activator inhibitor-1 in healthy middle-aged men. Arterioscler Thromb Vasc Biol 1996;16:363–7.

[95] Keltikangas-Jarvinen L, Raikkonen K, Hautanen A, et al. Vital exhaustion, anger expression, and pituitary and adrenocortical hormones: implications for the insulin resistance syndrome. Arterioscler Thromb Vasc Biol 1996;16:275–80.

[96] Nosadini R, Del Prato S, Tiengo A, et al. Insulin resistance in Cushing's syndrome. J Clin Endocrinol Metab 1983;57:529–36.

[97] Karnieli E, Cohen P, Barzilai N, Ish-Shalom Z, et al. Insulin resistance in Cushing's syndrome. Horm Metab Res 1985;17:518–21.

[98] Strasser RH, Braun-Dullaeus R, Walendzik H, et al. Alpha 1-receptor-independent activation of protein kinase C in acute myocardial ischemia: mechanisms for sensitization of the adenylyl cyclase system. Circ Res 1992;70:1304–12.

[99] di Paolo S, de Pergola G, Cospite MR, et al. Beta-adrenoceptors desensitization may modulate catecholamine induced insulin resistance in human pheochromocytoma. Diabetes Metab 1989;15:409–15.

[100] Raza SA, DeWitt RT, Chen H, et al. Catecholamine excess in pheochromocytoma inducing insulin resistance. Endocr Pract 2004;10:149–52.

[101] Wiesner TD, Bluher M, Windgassen M, et al. Improvement of insulin sensitivity after adrenalectomy in patients with pheochromocytoma. J Clin Endocrinol Metab 2003;88:3632–6.

[102] Bluher M, Windgassen M, Paschke R. Improvement of insulin sensitivity after adrenalectomy in patients with pheochromocytoma. Diabetes Care 2000;23:1591–2.

[103] Brunner EJ, Hemingway H, Walker BR, et al. Adrenocortical, autonomic, and inflammatory causes of the metabolic syndrome: nested case-control study. Circulation 2002;106:2659–65.

[104] Seematter G, Binnert C, Martin JL, et al. Relationship between stress, inflammation and metabolism. Curr Opin Clin Nutr Metab Care 2004;7:169–73.

[105] Rotter V, Nagaev I, Smith U. Interleukin-6 (IL-6) induces insulin resistance in 3T3–L1 adipocytes and is, like IL-8 and tumor necrosis factor-alpha, overexpressed in human fat cells from insulin-resistant subjects. J Biol Chem 2003;278:45777–84.

[106] Senn JJ, Klover PJ, Nowak IA, et al. Interleukin-6 induces cellular insulin resistance in hepatocytes. Diabetes 2002;51:3391–9.

[107] Pickup JC, Mattock MB, Chusney GD, et al. NIDDM as a disease of the innate immune system: association of acute-phase reactants and interleukin-6 with metabolic syndrome X. Diabetologia 1997;40:1286–92.

[108] Erren M, Reinecke H, Junker R, et al. Systemic inflammatory parameters in patients with atherosclerosis of the coronary and peripheral arteries. Arterioscler Thromb Vasc Biol 1999;19: 2355–63.

[109] Ridker PM, Rifai N, Stampfer MJ, et al. Plasma concentration of interleukin-6 and the risk of future myocardial infarction among apparently healthy men. Circulation 2000;101:1767–72.

[110] Schmidt AM, Hofmann M, Taguchi A, et al. RAGE: a multiligand receptor contributing to the cellular response in diabetic vasculopathy and inflammation. Semin Thromb Hemost 2000;26: 485–93.

[111] Schmidt AM, Stern DM. Receptor for age (RAGE) is a gene within the major histocompatibility class III region: implications for host response mechanisms in homeostasis and chronic disease. Front Biosci 2001;6:D1151–60.

[112] Schmidt AM, Yan SD, Yan SF, et al. The biology of the receptor for advanced glycation end products and its ligands. Biochim Biophys Acta 2000;1498:99–111.

[113] Bierhaus A, Humpert PM, Morcos M, et al. Understanding RAGE, the receptor for advanced glycation end products. J Mol Med 2005;83:876–86.

[114] Harbuz MS, Chover-Gonzalez AJ, Jessop DS. Hypothalamo-pituitary-adrenal axis and chronic immune activation. Ann N Y Acad Sci 2003;992:99–106.

[115] Jessop DS, Richards LJ, Harbuz MS. Effects of stress on inflammatory autoimmune disease: destructive or protective? Stress 2004;7:261–6.

[116] Straub RH, Dhabhar FS, Bijlsma JW, et al. How psychological stress via hormones and nerve fibers may exacerbate rheumatoid arthritis. Arthritis Rheum 2005;52:16–26.

[117] Carpeggiani C, Emdin M, Bonaguidi F, et al. Personality traits and heart rate variability predict long-term cardiac mortality after myocardial infarction. Eur Heart J 2005;26:1612–7.

[118] Tsuji H, Larson MG, Venditti Jr FJ, et al. Impact of reduced heart rate variability on risk for cardiac events: the Framingham Heart Study. Circulation 1996;94:2850–5.

[119] Maser RE, Mitchell BD, Vinik AI, et al. The association between cardiovascular autonomic neuropathy and mortality in individuals with diabetes: a meta-analysis. Diabetes Care 2003;26:1895–901.

[120] Vinik AI, Maser RE, Mitchell BD, et al. Diabetic autonomic neuropathy. Diabetes Care 2003;26:1553–79.

[121] Hayano J, Yamada A, Mukai S, et al. Severity of coronary atherosclerosis correlates with the respiratory component of heart rate variability. Am Heart J 1991;121:1070–9.

[122] Gianaros PJ, Salomon K, Zhou F, et al. A greater reduction in high-frequency heart rate variability to a psychological stressor is associated with subclinical coronary and aortic calcification in postmenopausal women. Psychosom Med 2005;67:553–60.

[123] Bierhaus A, Zhang Y, Deng Y, et al. Mechanism of the tumor necrosis factor alpha-mediated induction of endothelial tissue factor. J Biol Chem 1995;270:26419–32.

[124] Bierhaus A, Chen J, Liliensiek B, et al. LPS and cytokine activated endothelium. Semin Thromb Hemost 2000;26:571–88.

ANESTHESIOLOGY
CLINICS OF
NORTH AMERICA

ELSEVIER
SAUNDERS

Anesthesiology Clin N Am
24 (2006) 341–364

Novel Chemical Mediators in the Resolution of Inflammation: Resolvins and Protectins

Charles N. Serhan, PhD

Center for Experimental Therapeutics and Reperfusion Injury, Department of Anesthesiology,
Perioperative and Pain Medicine, Brigham and Women's Hospital and Harvard Medical School,
75 Francis Street, Boston, MA 02115, USA

The molecular basis for the beneficial impact of omega-3 fatty acids eicosapentaenoic acid (EPA) and docosahexaenoic acid (DHA) remains of interest. Recently, the author's laboratory identified novel local mediators generated from omega-3 essential fatty acids that displayed potent bioactions identified first in resolving inflammatory exudates and then in tissues enriched with DHA. The family names "resolvins" (resolution phase interaction products) and "protectins" were introduced for these two new families of bioactive compounds because they possess potent (on submicromolar-nanomolar levels) anti-inflammatory, immunoregulatory neuroprotective, and pro-resolving actions. The mediators derived from eicosapentaenoic acid that carry potent biological actions are designated E series (resolvins of the E series, ie, resolvin E1 [RvE1]), and those biosynthesized from the precursor DHA are denoted resolvins of the D series (ie, resolvin D1 [RvD1]). The bioactive compounds derived from DHA carrying conjugated triene structures (ie, docosatrienes) that possess immunoregulatory actions were termed protectins, and when they were generated within neural tissues, the preferred tissue/organ location is introduced in the trivial name "neuroprotectins" (NPD1). Aspirin treatment initiates a related epimeric series from each family by triggering the endogenous formation of the 17R series resolvins and protectins. These epimers were named aspirin-triggered (AT)-RvDs and protectins and possess potent anti-inflammatory actions in vivo, essentially equivalent to those evoked by their 17S series counterparts.

This work was supported in part by National Institutes of Health grants GM38675 and DK074448.
E-mail address: cnserhan@zeus.bwh.harvard.edu

342 SERHAN

This article provides an overview of these newly uncovered pathways and their potent bioaction products and focuses on their roles in the resolution of acute inflammation. Together, the activation of these biochemical pathways and their signaling demonstrate that resolution is an active programmed series of events initiated at the tissue/organ level with the onset of the host's response. This arena also provides previously unappreciated targets and approaches for the development of novel therapeutic interventions.

The essential role of dietary omega-3 polyunsaturated fatty acids (ω-3 PUFA) was uncovered in the late 1920s [1], and the importance of ω-3 PUFA was observed consistently for the remainder of the century [2–5]. In more recent studies, inflammation has emerged as a central component contributing to many prevalent diseases in modern Western civilization that were previously unknown to involve inflammation, including Alzheimer's disease, cardiovascular disease [6], and cancer [7,8], in addition to those that are associated with inflammation such as arthritis and periodontal disease [9,10]. In an effort to determine a link between omega-3 fatty acids and endogenous anti-inflammation, the present author and colleagues identified novel, enzymatically formed oxygenated products generated from the major ω-3 PUFA, EPA and DHA, which serve as precursors to the compounds that possess potent actions within resolving inflammatory exudates [11–15]. The names resolvins and protectins were introduced from initial studies because the new compounds displayed both potent anti-inflammatory and immunoregulatory properties.

This overview of the novel compounds and biosynthetic pathways from EPA and DHA that carry potent biological actions, the E series resolvins (resolvin E1 or RvE1) and D series (resolvin D1 or RvD1), as well as bioactive members from DHA carrying conjugated triene structures (docosatrienes), called protectins, that are both anti-inflammatory [12,13] and neuroprotective [14,15] and, when generated from neural tissues, termed neuroprotectins (NPD1) [15]. Other compounds identified earlier from omega-3 fatty acids have structures similar to eicosanoids but are less potent or completely devoid of apparent bioactivity, in sharp contrast to the resolvins and protectins, which evoke potent biological actions in vivo [11–15]. The resolvins and protectins are potent agonists of endogenous anti-inflammation and are pro-resolving chemical mediators.

When to resolve: a programmed series of events

The signs of inflammation (edema, redness, and heat) were already known to early civilizations. Egyptian hieroglyphics and ancient Greek and Chinese medical texts speak about the flame of inflammation and describe it, mistakenly, as a disease unto itself [16]. In 1794, the Scottish surgeon John Hunter wrote that "Inflammation in itself is not to be considered as a disease, but as a salutary operation consequent to some violence or some disease" [16]. His insight can be traced directly to our present appreciation of inflammation as a life-saving reaction; yet, this vital reaction is also associated with many of today's widespread diseases of Western cultures and unknown previously to be involved in the cause of cardiovascular disease, asthma, or Alzheimer's disease [17–19]. Dale of England [20] and von Euler of Sweden [21] each focused their seminal investigations on the roles of chemical mediators as short-range signals or autacoids in regulating cellular and tissue responses in neural systems. The role of chemical mediators in inflammation became apparent with the isolation of the prostaglandins, named by von Euler, and the discovery of the leukotrienes [22]. Although the contributions of phagocytes in host defense was described in the early studies of Metchnikoff [23], the lipid mediators generated by phagocytes, including neutrophils, monocytes and macrophages, are still evolving, given the intricate roles of these cell types [24] in the progression, duration, and termination of inflammatory responses.

There are many local, short-acting chemical mediators serving in pro-inflammatory roles that are produced initially while granulocytes approach microbes to be neutralized. From the early studies of Borgeat and Samuelsson [25], it became clear that neutrophils, when encountering materials to devour after they exit the post-capillary venules (Fig. 1), release mediators derived from arachidonic acid through cyclooxygenase and lipoxygenases that are, for the most part, pro-inflammatory (see Figs. 1 and 2A). One such chemical mediator is leukotriene B_4, a potent chemoattractant involved in the recruitment of additional neutrophils and leukocytes to the initial area of insult. Chemoattractants such as leukotriene B_4 work in concert with peptide chemoattractants (ie, chemokines and cytokines) [26,27] and are enhanced in many inflammatory diseases and therefore are the targets of many pharmaceutical companies' quests to control inflammation and minimize unwanted side effects that plague many current therapies. Because there are so many pro-inflammatory signals governing the vitality of the amplification phase [9], from the initial host-defense response to microbes, surgical trauma, or injury from within (see Fig. 1), searching for key regulators to control the excessive trafficking or aberrant activation of leukocytes is a paramount task. This dual mask of the effector response of neutrophils is well appreciated [26]. As primary defenders, neutrophils are able to congregate swiftly in large numbers yet can inadvertently spill noxious agents intended to kill or neutralize invaders, which in turn can evoke tissue damage and local inflammatory sequelae. The uncovering of novel endogenous mediators of anti-inflammation that control or dampen inflammation to keep it self-limited and promote resolution has raised awareness of the potential for new therapeutic approaches to inflammatory diseases that target these active pathways [27–30] and potentially to mechanisms underlying the basis of essential ω-3 PUFA deficiencies in humans.

Alpha signaling omega: switching eicosanoid classes and families of lipid mediators to resolve

An informatics liquid chromatography-tandem mass spectrometry (LC-MS-MS)-based approach was used in systematic studies of lipid mediators within the course

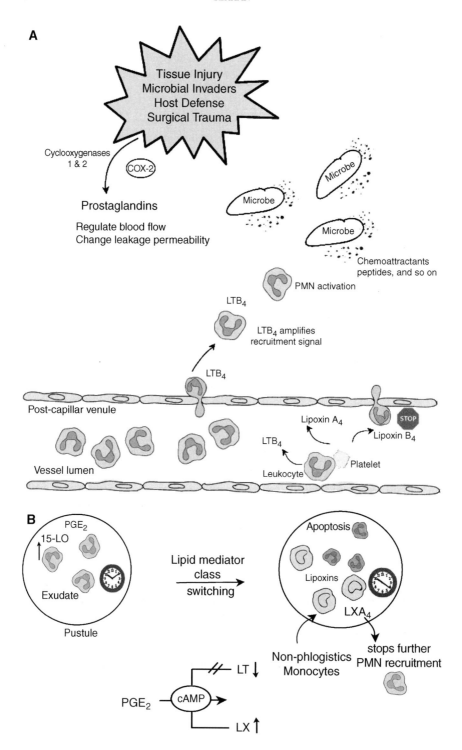

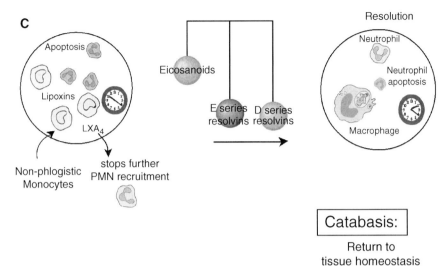

Fig. 1. Programmed temporal events in resolution of acute inflammation: the role of lipid-derived mediators. (A) Microbial invaders, tissue injury, and surgical trauma activate the release and formation of arachidonate-derived prostaglandins, which regulate early events in inflammatory response. Initial chemoattractants recruit PMNs that undergo diapedesis from postcapillary venules, an event that is amplified by the production of the 5-lipoxygenase pathway product leukotriene B$_4$, a potent chemoattractant (see text for details). During the progression of inflammatory events, platelet-leukocyte interactions evoke the formation of lipoxins A$_4$ and B$_4$, which serve as stop signals by blocking further recruitment of PMNs from the postcapillary venules. This strategic location limits the number of neutrophils required to combat microbes or to clean up tissue debris. (B) At contained sites of inflammation, as exudates form and pustules are walled off, prostaglandins initiate a number of responses relevant in inflammatory events, but most interestingly they signal the end by activating the transcriptional regulation of 15-LOX in neutrophils, which in turn leads to the temporal dissociation and production of lipoxins from arachidonic acid, which play pro-resolving and anti-inflammatory roles (see text for details). This is referred to as class switching within the arachidonic acid-derived eicosanoids from prostaglandins and leukotrienes to lipoxins that initiate or are coincident with the termination sequence at the tissue level. This stops further neutrophil entry into the exudate. (C) The reduction in PMN in the exudate is also temporally associated with a switch of the families of lipid mediators generated from eicosanoids to resolvins of the E and D series as well as protectins (see text for further details). The clock face illustrates the timeline for individual neutrophils and their set points as new neutrophils parachute into exudates. Note that exudate leukocytes are asynchronous.

of acute inflammatory responses [31]. During the initial phase (see Fig. 1A), prostaglandins (PG) such as PGE$_2$ are generated [33], which are involved in the early steps of the control of blood flow and vessel dilation needed for leukocytes to undergo firm adhesion and diapedesis [34,35]. The required traffic from the post-capillary lumen to the interstitial space is a process that is, in part, governed by leukotriene B$_4$ [35]. Programmed within this initial phase, there is also the activation of signaling pathways for the normal self-limiting or termination at local contained sites of inflammation [11,12,32]. Signaling pathways [36] leading to prostaglandin E$_2$ and D$_2$ in turn actively switch on production at the transcriptional level of enzymes required for the generation of another class of eicosanoids that are also

A

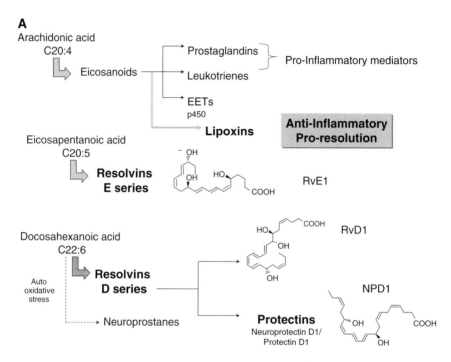

Fig. 2. The role of essential polyunsaturated fatty acids as precursors in the production of families of lipid mediators. (*A*) Precursors of lipid mediators: arachidonic acid is the precursor to eicosanoids that have distinct roles as proinflammatory mediators. The prostaglandins and leukotrienes each play specific actions pivotal to the progression of inflammation [101–103]. Arachidonic acid-derived epoxyeicosatetraenoic acids (EETs) produced through P450s also appear to play roles [104,105]. Cell-cell interactions, exemplified by platelet leukocytes within the vasculature or PMN-mucosal interactions, enhance generation of lipoxins that serve as intravascular stop signals and promote resolution, serving as endogenous anti-inflammatory mediators self-limiting the course of inflammation. The essential omega-3 fatty acids eicosapentaenoic acid and docosahexaenoic acid (C20:5 and C22:6) are converted to two novel families of lipid mediators, resolvins and protectins, that play pivotal roles in promoting resolution (see text for details). Resolvin E series are generated from eicosapentaenoic acid such as RvE1, and resolvins of the D series, such as resolvin D1, are generated from DHA as well as the protectins such as neuroprotectin D1 from DHA, which is enriched in neural systems [13–15]. (*B*) Aspirin triggering of lipid mediators: aspirin affects the formation of resolvin E1 by acetylating COX-2 in vascular endothelial cells that stereo-selectively can generate 18*R*-H(p)EPE that is picked up through transcellular metabolism by leukocytes and converted in a lipoxygenase-like mechanism to RvE1. The complete stereochemistries of RvE1 and one of its receptors were recently identified (see Fig. 5) [46]. Of interest, biosynthesis of RvE1 can also be initiated by P450-like enzymes in microbes [11]. Aspirin also affects the formation of D series resolvins and catalytically switches COX-2 to a 17*R*-lipoxygenase-like mechanism that generates 17*R*-series resolvin D. Aspirin affects the formation of protectins, and specifically neuroprotectin D1, through a similar mechanism that generates compounds carrying the 17*R* epimer at the carbon 17 position (see text and Figs. 5 and 6).

B

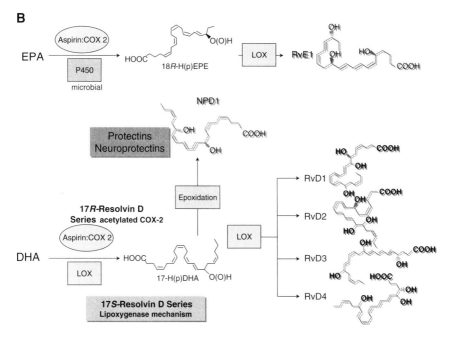

Fig. 2 (*continued*).

generated from arachidonic acid, such as lipoxins (LX) [32], and the novel families of lipid mediators, resolvins and protectins [11–14,24] generated from ω-3 PUFA that signal for resolution in this phase of the tissue response (Fig. 2; see also Fig. 1).

The lipoxins are now appreciated widely for their ability to actively promote resolution by regulating the entry of new neutrophils to sites of inflammation [37] and organs of reperfusion injury [38]; they reduce vascular permeability [39] while also stimulating the nonphlogistic infiltration of monocytes [29] that appear to be required for wound healing [40] and stimulate macrophages to uptake apoptotic neutrophils [41] (see Fig. 1B). This temporal switch in lipid mediator class within the family of eicosanoids (see Fig. 2) from pro- to anti-inflammatory eicosanoids (ie, PG and leukotriene [LT] progressing to LX) is an active process and also underscores the ability of leukocytes to trigger the self-limited response of acute inflammation [32]. This switch in lipid mediator classes also appears to be linked to a change in the phenotype and to the internal cellular clock of individual neutrophils within the site of inflammation (eg, within pustules [see Fig. 1]). Once a neutrophil jumps into an exudate, it can, by interacting with cells in the immediate environment (ie, other leukocytes, blood-borne cell types, platelets, endothelia, mucosal epithelia [42] or interstitial cells, and fibroblasts), undergo transcellular biosynthesis and switch its lipid mediator profile from, for example, leukotriene biosynthesis to lipoxin biosynthesis [32]. This initiation of the termination sequence in the early steps of the phagocytes' response appears to be a circuit that is used at the extracellular chemical mediator level as well as the intracellular signaling events through nuclear factor (NF)κB [43]. Hence, the beginning (alpha) signals the end (omega) of inflammation with the initiation governed by arachidonic acid-derived mediators that turn to the use of ω-3 PUFA in this process to generate resolvins and protectins (see below).

Spontaneous resolution milieu for the identification of resolvins and protectins

During the course of acute inflammatory response, mediators not only switch classes but also substrates to form novel families of chemical mediators [44]. The air pouch, which has been well studied by Perretti and Getting [45], undergoes spontaneous resolution. A systematic analysis of this phase, using a lipidomic or lipid mediator informatic approach with LC-MS-MS, revealed that during the time course of spontaneous resolution, novel lipid mediators were generated that were previously unknown. These resolution phase mediators were shown to use ω-3 PUFA (DHA and EPA) as substrates and are agonists for promoting resolution by stopping the further recruitment of leukocytes. The first of these are resolvins of the E series, which are biosynthesized from the precursor EPA [11,12,46].

Omega-3 PUFA have long been known [1] to play an essential role in maintaining organ function and health. Many clinical reports emphasize the importance of omega-3 supplementation in correcting disease-mediated events. Until the Gruppo Italiano per lo Studio della Sopravvivenza nell'Infarto Miocardioco (GISSI)-Prevenzione studies [2,47,48], the impact of omega-3's in many diseases remained unclear. Importantly, the roles of ω-3 PUFA, such as EPA and DHA, at the molecular level were the subject of much debate. The major mechanism of action for omega-3's was believed to block formation of pro-inflammatory mediators through substrate competition [2]. In sharp contrast, the present author and colleagues have found that during the course of inflammation and its active resolution, ω-3 PUFAs are used to generate novel lipid mediators that are agonists in anti-inflammation. Systematic analysis undertaken to define the indices of resolution using a combined trafficking proteomic and lipidomic approach revealed that representatives for each family of lipid mediators (LXA$_4$, RvE1, and neuroprotectin D1/protectin D1) (see Fig. 2A) act at different steps or points within the resolution indices recently defined [44]. Each compound is anti-inflammatory when given in vivo but, more importantly, can promote resolution by shortening the time interval or time for catabasis and the return of involved tissue to homeostasis [44].

The resolution of acute inflammation specifically involves mobilization of different fatty acid precursors that appear within exudates, arachidonic acid, EPA, and DHA in a temporally orchestrated fashion (see Fig. 1). Each precursor in turn is transformed to separate families of bioactive compounds that serve as local chemical mediators [24], which has significant implications regarding the programming and circuitry of lipid mediators in resolution. They also raise the possibility that deficiencies in ω-3 PUFA substrates, as might be expected in dietary supplementation or deficiencies of EPA or DHA, may lead to inappropriate resolution. Such possibilities are being tested. Nonetheless, systematic temporal-spatial analyses of murine peritonitis demonstrate that there is a clear program of events in resolution and that cellular trafficking and clearance is regulated in an active fashion by lipid-derived [44] and protein-derived mediators, such as annexins [27,41]. Lipoxin A_4 and annexin-1 share the ability to regulate expedited uptake of apoptotic neutrophils by macrophages (see Fig. 1C). The identification of the resolvin E_1 receptor, its presence on leukocytes and dendritic cells, and the importance of these cell types in inflammatory responses underscores the communication between early initial events in lipid-mediated biosynthesis and their linking to cellular trafficking [46], as well as governance for inflammation, as in models of inflammatory bowel disease [49,50].

Mapping of the resolution phase of acute inflammatory responses appears to be organ-specific as to the temporal relationships between lipid mediator classes [32,44,51]. Well-established and widely used drugs affect resolution [36,52]. In this context, aspirin (which is well appreciated for its ability to inhibit the formation of lipid mediators such as prostaglandins) [22,53] actually triggers the generation of epimeric forms of arachidonic acid [54] as well as the newly identified EPA- and DHA-derived mediators [11–13] that demonstrate potent anti-inflammatory and pro-resolving actions. The epimeric forms of lipoxins, for example, also called aspirin-triggered 15-epi-lipoxins, share their actions in vitro and in vivo, as appears to be the case with EPA- and DHA-derived resolvins of the D series (17R-containing resolvins and protectins) [13,14]. There is also clear evidence that glucocorticoids enhance the uptake and the limitation of apoptotic neutrophils [27,41,55], a key step in the clearance or expedition of the return of the tissue to homeostasis (see Fig. 1C). This active process of catabasis appears to be programmed at the level of chemical mediators, including lipid mediator and protein mediator levels [44]. Their role is likely governing both intracellular and extracellular signaling events that are involved in dampening inflammation and promoting its resolution.

Because aspirin and glucocorticoids both affect resolution and share, in the case of lipoxin, a common site of action (the lipoxin A_4 receptor), it is possible that other widely used common drugs can affect resolution pathways. Also, potential deficiencies inherited or acquired in these pathways may present in the clinic as the chronic inflammatory diseases we appreciate today [24].

Use of polyunsaturated fatty acids (n-6 versus n-3) during resolution of acute inflammation

It had often been questioned whether essential fatty acids, such as the omega-3 EPA or DHA, are converted to potent lipid mediators, as is the case with arachidonic acid. In short, both DHA and EPA are important precursors; we now appreciate that intimate cell-cell interactions within vessel walls (ie, adherent platelets that are studded with polymorphonuclear neutrophil [PMN] cells) converge on the endothelium and can be visualized by intravital microscopy [56,57], and they promote transcellular lipid mediator biosynthesis [58–60]. During platelet-leukocyte interactions, arachidonic acid is converted to LX, which are generated to act as "stop" signals on PMN (see Fig. 1A) in the nM range through specific receptors we identified [61,62] and confirmed by others [63,64], and stimulated monocytes [40] and macrophages to promote resolution [41].

These forms of cell-cell interactions in the vasculature are impinged upon by aspirin [54,65]. Aspirin inhibits thromboxane production by platelets and prostacyclin biosynthesis in vascular endothelial cells [66,67]. During PMN-endothelial or PMN-epithelial interactions (see Fig. 1A), aspirin triggers the biosynthesis of 15-epi-lipoxins (ATL) [54]; both LX and ATL and their respective stable analogs are potent regulators of transendothelial and transepithelial migration of PMN across these cells and endothelial cell proliferation in vitro and in vivo [68–70]. Also, transgenic mice over-expressing the human LXA_4 receptor with myeloid-specific promoter display was found to reduce PMN infiltration in peritonitis and heightened sensitivity to LXA_4 and ATL [71]. Transgenic rabbits over-expressing 15-lipoxygenase (LOX) type I generate enhanced levels of lipoxins, have an enhanced anti-inflammatory status, and are protected from the inflammatory bone loss of periodontal disease [72]. Hence, the results of these studies have heightened our awareness that PMN, in addition to their host-defense position and the possibility that they can spill proinflammatory agents (see Fig. 2) [73] and mediators such as the classic eicosanoids, prostanoids, and leukotrienes [22,53], which amplify inflammatory responses, can also produce novel protective lipid mediators, which actively counter-regulate the inflammation (Fig. 3).

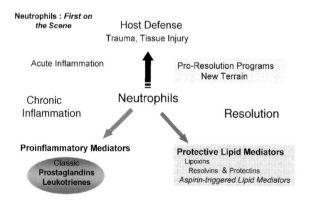

Fig. 3. Resolution phase role for neutrophils. PMN are first on the scene and can switch their phenotype to produce pro-resolving and protective lipid mediators during the evolution of the inflammatory exudate.

In view of the compelling results from the GISSI study showing improvements in >11,000 cardiovascular patients [47,48] (including reduction in sudden death by ~45% by receiving almost 1 g of omega-3 per day), a potential role of ω-3 PUFA was recently addressed. Inspection of the GISSI protocol indicated that all patients were also taking daily aspirin, which remained unaccounted for in their published analysis. Despite very large doses (in amounts of milligrams to grams daily), an abundant literature with omega (n-3) PUFA suggests beneficial actions in many human diseases, including periodontitis [74], anti-inflammatory, and antitumor actions [2,75]. Each of the three major human lipoxygenase activities (5-LOX, 12-LOX, and 15-LOX) can convert DHA to various monohydroxy-containing products; however, the in vivo functions of these LOX products were either not apparent or they did not display bioactivity [76,77]. DHA can also be non-enzymatically oxygenated to isoprostane-like compounds, termed neuroprostanes, that reflect oxidative stress in the brain [78] or auto-oxidized to products that are monohydroxy racemates [79] of the compounds that are now known to be enzymatically produced during biosynthesis of the resolvins and protectins [12–15]. Overall, it is noteworthy that the molecular and cellular mechanisms underlying omega-3's immunoprotective actions remains to be established, and their direct connection to human disease and treatment are biomedical challenges of importance [80].

The aspirin twist: aspirin-triggered lipid mediators

Aspirin is an active ingredient in >60 over-the-counter remedies, making it a difficult substance to control for rigorously in some human studies. In view of the aforementioned findings, the questions became apparent, namely, what is the molecular basis for omega n-3's protective action, and are there potential overlaps in their actions at the molecular and cellular levels? To address this in an experimental setting, the present author and colleagues used murine dorsal skin pouches [11,12], a model of inflammation known to resolve spontaneously in rats [81]. This model was adapted for mice to include both genetics and to set up lipidomics using liquid chromatography-ultraviolet-tandem mass spectrometry (LC-UV-MS-MS)-based analyses geared to evaluating whether potential novel lipid mediators were indeed generated during the resolution phase of inflammation [11,12]. In this pouch (experimental contained inflammation) after 4 hours, PMN numbers began to drop within exudates [11,12]. Exudates were taken at timed intervals, focusing on the period of "spontaneous resolution," and lipid mediator profiles were determined using tandem LC-UV-MS-MS. Lipid mediator libraries were constructed with physical properties (ie, MS and MS/MS spectra, elution times, UV spectra, and others) for matching and to assess whether known or potential novel lipid mediators were present within the exudates. These libraries and the software for matching them are presently expanding [31]. If novel lipid mediators were encountered, their structures were elucidated by carrying out retrograde analysis for both biogenic enzymatic synthesis and total organic synthesis. This approach permitted the assessment of structure-activity relationships as well as the scale-up required to confirm the bioactions of novel compounds identified [11,12,82].

18*R* E Series resolvins and 17*R* D series resolvins

Resolving exudates in mice contain 18*R*-HEPE as well as several related bioactive compounds [11]. These novel compounds are produced from EPA by at least one biosynthetic pathway operative in human cells. This pathway is illustrated in Figs. 2 and 4. Blood vessel-derived vascular endothelial cells treated with aspirin convert EPA to 18*R*-hydro(peroxy)-EPE, which is reduced to 18*R*-HEPE. This conversion is enhanced by hypoxia. The 18*R*-HEPE is released from endothelium and rapidly converted by the activated human PMN in proximity, for example by adherent PMN that transform 18*R*-HEPE to a 5(6) epoxide-containing intermediate that is further transformed to the bioactive 5,12,18*R*-trihydroxy-EPE. This bioactive mediator was termed a resolvin, specifically RvE1, because it was identified in the resolution phase in mice, appeared as cell-cell interaction/transcellular biosynthetic products with isolated human cells, and, importantly, proved to be a potent regulator of PMN and inflamma-

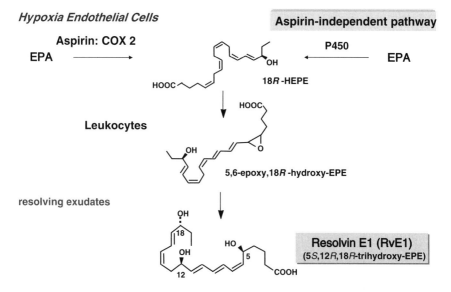

Fig. 4. Resolvin E1 biosynthesis from EPA; for example, human endothelial cells expressing COX-2 when treated with aspirin transform EPA. The mechanism involves abstracting hydrogen at carbon 16 in EPA to give *R* insertion of molecular oxygen, yielding 18*R*-hydroperoxy-EPE, which is reduced to 18*R*-HEPE. They can be further converted through sequential actions of leukocyte 5-LOX and lead to formation of the trihydroxy bioactive product 5,12,18*R*-triHEPE, termed resolvin E1 [12]. The recently established [46] complete stereochemistry of RvE1 is 5*S*,12*R*,18*R*-trihydroxy-6*Z*, 8*E*,10*E*,14*Z*,16*E*-eicosapentaenoic acid; one of its receptors was identified as a GPCR (see text).

tion (see Figs. 3 and 4). In the absence of aspirin, 18R-HEPE can be produced through a P450-like mechanism and by microbes [83,84]. Total organic synthesis of this compound as well as related isomers was achieved, and its complete stereochemical assignment was established as 5S,12R,18R-trihydroxy-6Z,8E,10E,14Z,16E-eicosapentaenoic acid [46].

In resolving exudates from mice given aspirin and DHA, novel 17R-hydroxy-docosahexaenoic acid (17R-HDHA) and several related bioactive compounds were identified (Fig. 5). Human microvascular endothelial cells, also aspirin-treated in hypoxia, generate 17R-HDHA. DHA is converted by human recombinant cyclooxygenase (COX)-2, which was surprising, because earlier literature indicated that DHA is not a substrate of cyclooxygenase [85,86]. However, these investigations were performed before knowledge about the COX-2 isoform, and they used organs rich in COX-1. Human recombinant COX-2 converts DHA to 13-hydroxy-DHA. With aspirin, this switches to 17R-oxygenation to

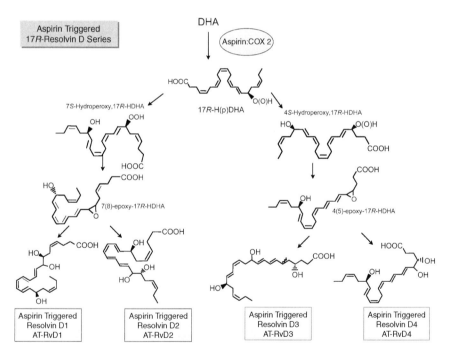

Fig. 5. Aspirin-triggered D series resolvins. The 17R series resolvins are produced from DHA in the presence of aspirin. Human endothelial cells expressing COX-2 treated with aspirin transform DHA to 17R-HDHA. Human PMN convert 17R-HDHA to two compounds through 5-lipoxygenation (modeled with the potato 5LO) [11,12] that are each rapidly transformed into two epoxide intermediates: a 7(8)-epoxide (left side) and the other a 4(5)-epoxide. These two novel epoxide intermediates can be enzymatically opened to bioactive products denoted 17R series ATRvD1 through ATRvD6. Note, the stereochemistry is shown in its likely configuration based on results with recombinant enzymes [12,13]. The total synthesis of RvD was recently reported [106].

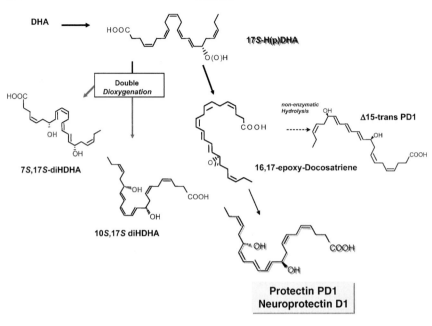

Fig. 6. Protectin biosynthesis and neuroprotectin D1/protectin D1 pathway. Formed from DHA, the lipoxygenase product 17S-H(p)DHA is converted to a 16(17)-epoxide that is enzymatically converted to the 10,17-dihydroxy bioactive product [13], denoted earlier as 10,17S-docosatriene (DT) [14] and recently called neuroprotectin D1/protectin D1, based on its potent actions in vivo [14,15]. The complete stereochemistry was recently established. The pathways are shown in their determined configurations with related biosynthetic isomers.

give epimeric AT forms (also in brain) [12,13] of both resolvins (RvD1–RvD4) and protectins (Fig. 6; see also Fig. 5).

17S D Series resolvins

Using lipid mediator informatics and LC-MS-MS-based analyses, the present author and colleagues learned that without aspirin or added DHA, the endogenous DHA was converted in vivo to a 17S series of resolvins (RvD1–RvD4) as well as docosatriene (DT) (such as 10,17S-DT) [13,14]. As in most structural elucidation experiments, added substrates were used to confirm biosynthesis and to isolate quantities of the novel active principle for bioassay. In this case, given the large doses in humans, experimental animals, and in vitro cell culture studies needed to observe the effects in omega-3 supplement studies [2–5], it was expected that these precursors (ie, EPA and DHA) needed to be added in the present studies. This proved not to be the case. Tissues such as normal mouse tissue and isolated human neural cells contain DHA that is available on activation to pro-

Table 1
Actions of resolvins and protectins

Mediator	Action	Study
Resolvin E1	Reduces PMN infiltration, murine skin air pouch inflammation, peritonitis	Serhan et al, 2000 [11]; Serhan et al, 2002 [12]; Arita et al 2005 [46]; Bannenberg et al, 2005 [44]
	Gastrointestinal protection in TNBS colitis	Arita et al, 2005 [49]
	Protects in periodontitis, stops inflammation and bone loss	Hasturk et al, 2006 [88]
Resolvin D1	Reduces PMN infiltration, murine skin air pouch inflammation	Serhan et al, 2002 [12]
	Reduces peritonitis	Hong et al, 2003 [13]
	Reduces cytokine expression in microglial cells	Hong et al, 2003 [13]
	Protects in renal ischemic injury	Duffield et al, in press [89]
Protectin D1/ neuroprotectin D1	Reduces stroke damage	Marcheselli et al, 2003 [14]
	Reduces PMN infiltration	Hong et al, 2003 [13]
	Protects from retinal injury	Mukherjee et al, 2004 [15]
	Regulates T_H2 cells, apoptosis and raft formation	Ariel et al, 2005 [90]
	Shortens resolution interval in murine peritonitis; regulates cytokines and chemokines	Bannenberg et al, 2005 [44]
Protectin D1/ neuroprotectin D1	Reduces PMN infiltration; reduces peritonitis	Serhan et al, 2006 [82]
	Diminished production in human Alzheimer disease and promotes neural cell survival	Lukiw et al, 2005 [91]
	Promotes corneal epithelial cell wound healing	Gronert et al, 2005 [87]

Abbreviation: T_H, T-helper.

duce 17*S*-containing DT and RvDs in vivo [11–15] with potent bioactions (Table 1) [11–15,44,46,49,82–91].

Endogenous anti-inflammation and pro-resolving biosynthetic pathways: microbes in the mix

With microglial cells that liberate cytokines in the brain, the D class resolvins block tumor necrosis factor (TNF)-α-induced interleukin (IL)-1β transcripts and are potent regulators of PMN infiltration in brain, skin, and peritonitis in vivo [13,14]. Of the docosatriene or protectin family, 10,17*S*-DT, the neuroprotectin D1/protectin D1 pathway (see Fig. 6) proved to be a potent regulator of PMN influx in exudates, at sites where it is formed from endogenous precursors [12,13], limiting stroke brain injury [14] and retinal pigmented cellular damage [15]. Other dihydroxy-docosanoids were less active in these bioassay settings [13,15].

Direct comparisons between resolvin E class versus the D classes (17R and 17S epimer series) for their ability to regulate PMN in vivo were performed [12,13,72]. Both the D and E classes of Rv are potent regulators of PMN infiltration. RvD class 17R series, triggered by aspirin, and the 17S series give essentially similar results (DHA-derived trihydroxy resolvins), indicating that the S-to-R switch does not diminish their bioactions. When injected intravenously, 100 ng/mouse, they both gave ~50% inhibition, and the RvE1 gave ~75% to 80% inhibition. In comparison, indomethacin at 100 ng/mouse (or ~3 µg/kg) gave roughly 25% inhibition [12,13].

The main bioactive resolvins and protectins as representative members are shown in Figs. 2 through 6. The formation of these compounds may involve enzymes that are also known to convert arachidonic acid as substrate. Because it is possible that, in view of the many lipoxygenases identified to date with unknown functions or specific polyunsaturated fatty acids as substrates [92,93], strategically positioned enzymes may be specifically involved in pathways that produce these novel compounds. Generally, lipoxygenases are defined by their ability to convert polyunsaturated fatty acids that contain cis,cis-1,4-pentadiene subunits to hydroperoxy-containing products that can serve as intermediates (Fig. 7). A well-appreciated substrate in human tissues is arachidonic acid; the main lipoxygenases convert arachidonic acid to the corresponding 5S-, 12S-, or 15S-hydroperoxyeicosatetraenoic acids. Hence, these enzymes came to be known as the arachidonate:oxygen 5-oxidoreductase (5-LOX), arachidonate:oxygen

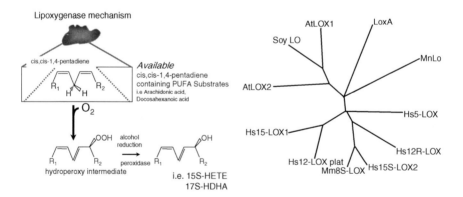

Fig. 7. General mechanism of lipoxygenases with molecular oxygen. The dendogram at right shows the diversity in different animal and plant lipoxygenases. The following lipoxygenase sequences were aligned using Clustal X (SGI, Mountain View, California) software (GenBank accession numbers are indicated): LoxA (*Pseudomonas aeruginosa* lipoxygenase, PA1169/A83499); MnLo (*Gaeumannomyces graminis* manganese lipoxygenase, AY040824); Hs5-LOX (*Homo sapiens* 5-lipoxygenase, P09917); Hs12R-LOX (*Homo sapiens* 12R-lipoxygenase, AF038461); Hs15S-LOX2 (*Homo sapiens* 15S-lipoxygenase type 2, NM_001141); Mm8S-LOX (*Mus musculus* 8S-lipoxygenase, U93277); Hs12-LOX plat (*Homo sapiens* platelet 12-lipoxygenase, P18054); Hs15-LOX1 (*Homo sapiens* 15-lipoxygenase type I, M23892); AtLOX2 (*Arabidopsis thaliana* lipoxygenase 2, JQ2391); soy LOX (soybean lipoxygenase 5, U50075); and AtLOX1 (*Arabidopsis thaliana* lipoxygenase 1, JQ2267). The alignment was used to construct this unrooted tree dendrogram [98].

12-oxidoreductase (12-LOX), and arachidonate:oxygen 15-oxidoreductase (15-LOX). The release and availability of substrate are critical to indicating the preferred substrate of a given lipoxygenase, which appears to be best appreciated only in the case of 5-lipoxygenase and leukotriene biosynthesis [94]. With the identification of lipoxygenase through molecular cloning, many additional lipoxygenases have been discovered, but their preferred substrates and role in vivo are not completely established. These include 12R-LOX, 15-LOX type 2, soluble 15-LOX (LoxA), and 8S-lipoxygenase (see Fig. 7). Each of these was cataloged according to its position of molecular insertion into arachidonate [95–98]. It follows that specific hydrolases, synthases, and related enzymes specialized to handle DHA- and EPA-derived intermediates are likely to be involved in these novel compounds and pathways. It remains to be established whether EPA and DHA are each converted by either specific pathways that biosynthesize these novel bioactive products or whether they simply commandeer the eicosanoid pathways as competitive substrates in these routes to generate the new bioactive products [13,87]. Along these lines, fish, which are abundant in ω-3 PUFA, biosynthesize these compounds, indicating that the resolvins and protectins are highly conserved structures [99].

Resolvins and protectins in disease models

Results from several recent studies indicate that resolvins and protectins have potent agonist actions that are of interest in managing human disease. The key points from these studies are summarized in Table 1. RvE1 was recently identified in human plasma [46]. At nanomolar levels, RvE1 dramatically reduced dermal inflammation, peritonitis, dendritic cell (DC) migration and IL-12 production. The present author and colleagues screened G protein-coupled receptors and identified one, denoted previously as the orphan GPCR ChemR23, which mediates RvE1 signal to attenuate NFκB. Specific binding of RvE1 to this receptor was confirmed using synthetic ^{3}H-labeled RvE1 that was prepared and isolated to confirm the specific interactions of RvE1 with ChemR23. Treatment of DCs with small-interfering RNA specific for ChemR23 sharply reduced RvE1 regulation of IL-12. These results demonstrated the novel counterregulatory responses in inflammation initiated through RvE1-receptor activation and provided the first evidence for EPA-derived potent endogenous agonists of anti-inflammation.

RvE1 (5S,12R,18R-trihydroxyeicosapentaenoic acid), as a synthetic anti-inflammatory lipid mediator, reduces leukocyte infiltration in several mouse disease models as well as in a rabbit model of periodontal disease (see Table 1). The administration of synthetic RvE1 blocks PMN infiltration in periodontal disease [88] and protects against the development of 2,4,6-trinitrobenzene sulfonic acid (TNBS)-induced colitis [49]. The beneficial action of RvE1 was quantified by increased survival rates, sustained body weight, improvement of histologic scores, reduced serum anti-TNBS IgG, decreased leukocyte infiltration and pro-inflammatory gene expression, including IL-12 p40, TNF-α, and iNOS. Thus, RvE1 counter-regulates in vivo leukocyte-mediated tissue injury and pro-inflammatory gene expression [44]. These findings show a novel endogenous mechanism that may underlie the beneficial actions of omega-3 EPA and provide new approaches for the treatment of gastrointestinal mucosal and oral inflammation.

Protectin D (PD)1 (*neuro*protectin D1 when generated by neural cells) was found to possess potent bioactions both in vivo and in vitro [1–3]. The complete stereochemistry of protectin D1 (10,17S-docosatriene), namely chirality of the carbon 10 alcohol and geometry of the conjugated triene required for bioactivity, remains to be established and was recently assigned. PD1 generated by human neutrophils during murine peritonitis and by neural tissues was separated from related natural isomers and was then subjected to LC-MS-MS and gas chromatography-mass spectrometry (GC-MS)-based analyses [82]. Comparison with six 10,17-dihydroxydocosatrienes prepared by total organic and biogenic synthesis showed that PD1, identified earlier from human cells (see Table 1), carries potent bioactivity; its complete stereochemistry is 10R,17S-dihydroxy-docosa-4Z,7Z,11E,13E,15Z,19Z-hexaenoic acid. Additional isomers identified in these studies include Δ15-*trans*-PD1 (isomer III), 10S,17S-dihydroxy-docosa-4Z,7Z,11E,13Z,15E,19Z-hexaenoic acid (isomer IV), and a double dioxygenation product, 10S,17S-dihydroxy-docosa-4Z,7Z,11E,13Z,15E,19Z-hexaenoic acid, that was also present in murine exudates. $^{18}O_2$ labeling showed that 10S,17S-diHDHA (isomer I) carried ^{18}O in the 10 position alcohol, indicating sequential lipoxygenation. This biosynthetic route is in sharp contrast to PD1 formation, which proceeds through an epoxide intermediate in situ and leads to the potent bioactive mediator. Synthetic PD1 at 10 nM attenuated (~50%) human neutrophil transmigration and its Δ15-*trans*-PD1 was essentially inactive. In addition, PD1 is a potent regulator of PMN infiltration (~40% at 1 ng/mouse) in peritonitis. The rank order at 1 to 10 ng per dose was PD1 ≈ PD1 methyl ester >> Δ15-*trans* PD1 >10S,17S-diHDHA (isomer I). Of interest to potential treatment roles for these new compounds, PD1 also reduced PMN infiltration after initiation (2 hours) of inflammation and was additive with resolvin E1. Together, these results indicate that PD1 is a potent stereoselective anti-inflammatory molecule [12,13,82]. Moreover, results of studies with Bazan and colleagues in neural tissues (see Table 1) and recently others indicate that PD1 also displays potent protective actions as well as wound healing capacity.

Summary

Resolvins and protectins are new families consisting of distinct chemical series of lipid-derived mediators, each with unique structures and apparent complementary anti-inflammatory actions. Both families of compounds, Rv and protectins, are also generated when aspirin is given in mammalian systems in their respective epimeric forms [11,12]. The resolvins and protectins each dampen inflammation and PMN-mediated injury from within, which is a key culprit in many common human diseases. The results of these initial studies underscore the roles of resolvins and protectins in inflammation resolution as well as catabasis and spotlight the therapeutic potential for this new arena of immunomodulation and host protection. It is likely that the resolvins, protectins, and their AT-related forms may play roles in other tissues and organs. Moreover, it is noteworthy that fish (eg, trout) generate lipoxygenase products such as LXA_5 from endogenous EPA [100] and also biosynthesize RvDs and protectins from endogenous DHA [99]. Taken together, these findings suggest that these novel lipid mediators (eg, resolvins and protectins) are conserved in evolution as self-protective and host-protective chemical mediators. In view of the essential roles of DHA and EPA in human biology and medicine uncovered to date [2–5,11], the physiologic relevance of the resolvins and protectins is likely to extend beyond our current appreciation [11–15].

Acknowledgments

The author thanks Mary Halm Small for expert assistance in preparing the manuscript.

References

[1] Burr GO, Burr MM. A new deficiency disease produced by the rigid exclusion of fat from the diet. J Biol Chem 1929;82:345–67.

[2] Lands WEM, editor. Proceedings of the American Oil Chemists' Society Short Course on Polyunsaturated Fatty Acids and Eicosanoids. Champaign (IL): American Oil Chemists' Society; 1987.

[3] Bazan NG. Supply of n-3 polyunsaturated fatty acids and their significance in the central nervous system. In: Wurtman RJ, Wurtman JJ, editors. Nutrition and the brain, volume 8. New York: Raven Press; 1990. p. 1–22.

[4] Simopoulos AP, Leaf A, Salem Jr N. Workshop on the essentiality of and recommended dietary intakes for omega-6 and omega-3 fatty acids. J Am Coll Nutr 1999;18:487–9.

[5] Salem Jr N, Litman B, Kim H-Y, et al. Mechanisms of action of docosahexaenoic acid in the nervous system. Lipids 2001;36:945–59.

[6] Helgadottir A, Manolescu A, Thorleifsson G, et al. The gene encoding 5-lipoxygenase activating protein confers risk of myocardial infarction and stroke. Nat Genet 2004;36: 233–9.

[7] Erlinger TP, Platz EA, Rifai N, et al. C-reactive protein and the risk of incident colorectal cancer. JAMA 2004;291:585–90.

[8] Pasche B, Serhan CN. Is C-reactive protein an inflammation opsonin that signals colon cancer risk? JAMA 2004;291:623–4.

[9] Gallin JI, Snyderman R, Fearon DT, et al, editors. Inflammation: basic principles and clinical correlates. 3rd edition. Philadelphia: Lippincott Williams & Wilkins; 1999. p. 1360.

[10] Van Dyke TE, Serhan CN. Resolution of inflammation: a new paradigm for the pathogenesis of periodontal diseases. J Dent Res 2003;82:82–90.

[11] Serhan CN, Clish CB, Brannon J, et al. Novel functional sets of lipid-derived mediators with antiinflammatory actions generated from omega-3 fatty acids via cyclooxygenase 2-nonsteroidal antiinflammatory drugs and transcellular processing. J Exp Med 2000;192: 1197–204.

[12] Serhan CN, Hong S, Gronert K, et al. Resolvins: a family of bioactive products of omega-3 fatty acid transformation circuits initiated by aspirin treatment that counter pro-inflammation signals. J Exp Med 2002;196:1025–37.

[13] Hong S, Gronert K, Devchand P, et al. Novel docosatrienes and 17S-resolvins generated from docosahexaenoic acid in murine brain, human blood and glial cells: autacoids in anti-inflammation. J Biol Chem 2003;278:14677–87.

[14] Marcheselli VL, Hong S, Lukiw WJ, et al. Novel docosanoids inhibit brain ischemia-reperfusion-mediated leukocyte infiltration and pro-inflammatory gene expression. J Biol Chem 2003;278:43807–17.

[15] Mukherjee PK, Marcheselli VL, Serhan CN, et al. Neuroprotectin D1: a docosahexaenoic acid-derived docosatriene protects human retinal pigment epithelial cells from oxidative stress. Proc Natl Acad Sci U S A 2004;101:8491–6.

[16] Majno G. The healing hand: man and wound in the ancient world. Cambridge (MA): Harvard University Press; 1975.

[17] Libby P. Atherosclerosis: the new view. Sci Am 2002;286:46–55.

[18] Drazen JM, Israel E, O'Byrne PM. Treatment of asthma with drugs modifying the leukotriene pathway. N Engl J Med 1999;340:197–206.

[19] Weiner HL, Selkoe DJ. Inflammation and therapeutic vaccination in CNS diseases. Nature 2002;420:879–84.

[20] Dale HH. Pharmacology during the past sixty years. In: Gibson WC, editor. The excitement and fascination of science: reflections by eminent scientists, vol. 1. Palo Alto (CA): Annual Reviews; 1978. p. 75.

[21] von Euler US. Pieces in the puzzle. In: Gibson WC, editor. The excitement and fascination of science: reflections by eminent scientists, vol. 2. Palo Alto (CA): Annual Reviews; 1978. p. 675–86.

[22] Samuelsson B. From studies of biochemical mechanisms to novel biological mediators: prostaglandin endoperoxides, thromboxanes and leukotrienes. In: The Nobel Foundation, editors. Les prix Nobel: Nobel prizes, presentations, biographies and lectures. Stockholm, Sweden: Almqvist & Wiksell; 1982. p. 153–74.

[23] Tauber AI, Chernyak L. Metchnikoff and the origins of immunology: from metaphor to theory. New York: Oxford University Press; 1991.

[24] Serhan CN. A search for endogenous mechanisms of anti-inflammation uncovers novel chemical mediators: missing links to resolution. Histochem Cell Biol 2004;122:305–21.

[25] Borgeat P, Samuelsson B. Arachidonic acid metabolism in polymorphonuclear leukocytes: effects of ionophore A23187. Proc Natl Acad Sci U S A 1979;76:2148–52.

[26] Cassatella MA, editor. Chemical Immunology and Allergy. The Neutrophil, vol 83. Basel, Switzerland: Karger; 2003.

[27] Gilroy DW, Perretti M. Aspirin and steroids: new mechanistic findings and avenues for drug discovery. Curr Opin Pharmacol 2005;5:405–11.

[28] Serhan CN. Lipoxin biosynthesis and its impact in inflammatory and vascular events. Biochim Biophys Acta 1994;1212:1–25.

[29] Lawrence T, Willoughby DA, Gilroy DW. Anti-inflammatory lipid mediators and insights into the resolution of inflammation. Nat Rev Immunol 2002;2:787–95.

[30] Nathan C. Points of control in inflammation. Nature 2002;420:846–52.

[31] Lu Y, Hong S, Tjonahen E, et al. Mediator-lipidomics: databases and search algorithms for PUFA-derived mediators. J Lipid Res 2005;46:790–802.

[32] Levy BD, Clish CB, Schmidt B, et al. Lipid mediator class switching during acute inflammation: signals in resolution. Nat Immunol 2001;2:612–9.

[33] Cotran RS, Kumar V, Collins T, editors. Robbins pathologic basis of disease. 6th edition. Philadelphia: WB Saunders; 1999. p. 1425.

[34] Williams TJ, Peck MJ. Role of prostaglandin-mediated vasodilatation in inflammation. Nature 1977;270:530–2.
[35] Pouliot M, Fiset ME, Masse M, et al. Adenosine up-regulates cyclooxygenase-2 in human granulocytes: impact on the balance of eicosanoid generation. J Immunol 2002;169: 5279–86.
[36] Gilroy DW, Colville-Nash PR, Willis D, et al. Inducible cyclooxygenase may have anti-inflammatory properties. Nat Med 1999;5:698–701.
[37] Serhan CN, Maddox JF, Petasis NA, et al. Design of lipoxin A$_4$ stable analogs that block transmigration and adhesion of human neutrophils. Biochemistry 1995;34:14609–15.
[38] Chiang N, Gronert K, Clish CB, et al. Leukotriene B$_4$ receptor transgenic mice reveal novel protective roles for lipoxins and aspirin-triggered lipoxins in reperfusion. J Clin Invest 1999; 104:309–16.
[39] Takano T, Clish CB, Gronert K, et al. Neutrophil-mediated changes in vascular permeability are inhibited by topical application of aspirin-triggered 15-epi-lipoxin A$_4$ and novel lipoxin B$_4$ stable analogues. J Clin Invest 1998;101:819–26.
[40] Maddox JF, Serhan CN. Lipoxin A$_4$ and B$_4$ are potent stimuli for human monocyte migration and adhesion: selective inactivation by dehydrogenation and reduction. J Exp Med 1996;183: 137–46.
[41] Godson C, Mitchell S, Harvey K, et al. Cutting edge: lipoxins rapidly stimulate nonphlogistic phagocytosis of apoptotic neutrophils by monocyte-derived macrophages. J Immunol 2000; 164:1663–7.
[42] Colgan SP, Serhan CN, Parkos CA, et al. Lipoxin A$_4$ modulates transmigration of human neutrophils across intestinal epithelial monolayers. J Clin Invest 1993;92:75–82.
[43] Lawrence T, Bebien M, Liu GY, et al. IKKalpha limits macrophage NF-kappaB activation and contributes to the resolution of inflammation. Nature 2005;434:1138–43.
[44] Bannenberg GL, Chiang N, Ariel A, et al. Molecular circuits of resolution: Formation and actions of resolvins and protectins. J Immunol 2005;174:4345–55.
[45] Perretti M, Getting SJ. Migration of specific leukocyte subsets in response to cytokine or chemokine application in vivo. In: Winyard PG, Willoughby DA, editors. Inflammation protocols, vol. 225. Totowa (NJ): Humana Press; 2003. p. 139–46.
[46] Arita M, Bianchini F, Aliberti J, et al. Stereochemical assignment, anti-inflammatory properties, and receptor for the omega-3 lipid mediator resolvin E1. J Exp Med 2005;201:713–22.
[47] GISSI-Prevenzione Investigators (Gruppo Italiano per lo Studio della Sopravvivenza nell'Infarto miocardico). Dietary supplementation with n-3 polyunsaturated fatty acids and vitamin E after myocardial infarction: results of the GISSI-Prevenzione trial. Lancet 1999; 354(9177):447–55.
[48] Marchioli R, Barzi F, Bomba E, et al. Early protection against sudden death by n-3 polyunsaturated fatty acids after myocardial infarction: time-course analysis of the results of the Gruppo Italiano per lo Studio della Sopravvivenza nell'Infarto Miocardico (GISSI)-Prevenzione. Circulation 2002;105:1897–903.
[49] Arita M, Yoshida M, Hong S, et al. Resolvin E1, a novel endogenous lipid mediator derived from omega-3 eicosapentaenoic acid, protects against TNBS-induced colitis. Proc Natl Acad Sci U S A 2005;102:7671–6.
[50] Wallace JL, Fiorucci S. A magic bullet for mucosal protection: and aspirin is the trigger! Trends Pharmacol Sci 2003;24:323–6.
[51] Fukunaga K, Kohli P, Bonnans C, et al. Cyclooxygenase 2 plays a pivotal role in the resolution of acute lung injury. J Immunol 2005;174:5033–9.
[52] Gilroy DW, Lawrence T, Perretti M, et al. Inflammation resolution: new opportunities for drug discovery. Nat Rev Drug Discov 2004;3:401–16.
[53] Vane JR. Adventures and excursions in bioassay: the stepping stones to prostacyclin. In: Les prix Nobel: Nobel prizes, presentations, biographies and lectures. Stockholm, Sweden: Almqvist & Wiksell; 1982. p. 181–206.
[54] Clària J, Serhan CN. Aspirin triggers previously undescribed bioactive eicosanoids by human endothelial cell-leukocyte interactions. Proc Natl Acad Sci U S A 1995;92:9475–9.

[55] Mitchell S, Thomas G, Harvey K, et al. Lipoxins, aspirin-triggered epi-lipoxins, lipoxin stable analogues, and the resolution of inflammation: stimulation of macrophage phagocytosis of apoptotic neutrophils in vivo. J Am Soc Nephrol 2002;13:2497–507.

[56] Lehr H-A, Olofsson AM, Carew TE, et al. P-selectin mediates the interaction of circulating leukocytes with platelets and microvascular endothelium in response to oxidized lipoprotein in vivo. Lab Invest 1994;71:380–6.

[57] Mora JR, Bono MR, Manjunath N, et al. Selective imprinting of gut-homing T cells by Peyer's patch dendritic cells. Nature 2003;424:88–93.

[58] Serhan CN, Hamberg M, Samuelsson B. Lipoxins: novel series of biologically active compounds formed from arachidonic acid in human leukocytes. Proc Natl Acad Sci U S A 1984; 81:5335–9.

[59] Serhan CN, Sheppard KA. Lipoxin formation during human neutrophil-platelet interactions: evidence for the transformation of leukotriene A_4 by platelet 12-lipoxygenase in vitro. J Clin Invest 1990;85:772–80.

[60] Marcus AJ. Platelets: their role in hemostasis, thrombosis, and inflammation. In: Gallin JI, Snyderman R, editors. Inflammation: basic principles and clinical correlates. Philadelphia: Lippincott Williams & Wilkins; 1999. p. 77–95.

[61] Fiore S, Ryeom SW, Weller PF, et al. Lipoxin recognition sites: specific binding of labeled lipoxin A_4 with human neutrophils. J Biol Chem 1992;267:16168–76.

[62] Fiore S, Maddox JF, Perez HD, et al. Identification of a human cDNA encoding a functional high affinity lipoxin A_4 receptor. J Exp Med 1994;180:253–60.

[63] Bae Y-S, Park JC, He R, et al. Differential signaling of formyl peptide receptor-like 1 by Trp-Lys-Tyr-Met-Val-Met-$CONH_2$ or lipoxin A_4 in human neutrophils. Mol Pharmacol 2003;63: 721–30.

[64] Gewirtz AT, Collier-Hyams LS, Young AN, et al. Lipoxin A_4 analogs attenuate induction of intestinal epithelial proinflammatory gene expression and reduce the severity of dextran sodium sulfate-induced colitis. J Immunol 2002;168:5260–7.

[65] Perretti M, Chiang N, La M, et al. Endogenous lipid- and peptide-derived anti-inflammatory pathways generated with glucocorticoid and aspirin treatment activate the lipoxin A(4) receptor. Nat Med 2002;8:1296–302.

[66] Vane JR. Back to an aspirin a day? Science 2002;296:474–5.

[67] Cheng Y, Austin SC, Rocca B, et al. Role of prostacyclin in the cardiovascular response to thromboxane A_2. Science 2002;296:539–41.

[68] Fierro IM, Colgan SP, Bernasconi G, et al. Lipoxin A_4 and aspirin-triggered 15-epi-lipoxin A_4 inhibit human neutrophil migration: comparisons between synthetic 15 epimers in chemotaxis and transmigration with microvessel endothelial cells and epithelial cells. J Immunol 2003;170: 2688–94.

[69] Fierro IM, Kutok JL, Serhan CN. Novel lipid mediator regulators of endothelial cell proliferation and migration: aspirin-triggered-15R-lipoxin A_4 and lipoxin A_4. J Pharmacol Exp Ther 2002;300:385–92.

[70] Kieran NE, Doran PP, Connolly SB, et al. Modification of the transcriptomic response to renal ischemia/reperfusion injury by lipoxin analog. Kidney Int 2003;64:480–92.

[71] Devchand PR, Arita M, Hong S, et al. Human ALX receptor regulates neutrophil recruitment in transgenic mice: Roles in inflammation and host-defense. FASEB J 2003;17:652–9.

[72] Serhan CN, Jain A, Marleau S, et al. Reduced inflammation and tissue damage in transgenic rabbits overexpressing 15-lipoxygenase and endogenous anti-inflammatory lipid mediators. J Immunol 2003;171:6856–65.

[73] Weissmann G, Smolen JE, Korchak HM. Release of inflammatory mediators from stimulated neutrophils. N Engl J Med 1980;303:27–34.

[74] Rosenstein ED, Kushner LJ, Kramer N, et al. Pilot study of dietary fatty acid supplementation in the treatment of adult periodontitis. Prostaglandins Leukot Essent Fatty Acids 2003;68: 213–8.

[75] Bazan NG. Supply, uptake, and utilization of docosahexaenoic acid during photoreceptor cell differentiation. Nestle Nutrition Workshop Series 1992;28:121–33.

[76] Lee TH, Mencia-Huerta J-M, Shih C, et al. Effects of exogenous arachidonic, eicosapen-taenoic, and docosahexaenoic acids on the generation of 5-lipoxygenase pathway products by ionophore-activated human neutrophils. J Clin Invest 1984;74:1922–33.

[77] Sawazaki S, Salem Jr N, Kim H-Y. Lipoxygenation of docosahexaenoic acid by the rat pineal body. J Neurochem 1994;62:2437–47.

[78] Reich EE, Zackert WE, Brame CJ, et al. Formation of novel D-ring and E-ring isoprostane-like compounds (D_4/E_4-neuroprostanes) in vivo from docosahexaenoic acid. Biochemistry 2000;39: 2376–83.

[79] VanRollins M, Baker RC, Sprecher HW, et al. Oxidation of docosahexaenoic acid by rat liver microsomes. J Biol Chem 1984;259:5776–83.

[80] Lands WEM. Diets could prevent many diseases. Lipids 2003;38:317–21.

[81] Winyard PG, Willoughby DA, editors. Methods in Molecular Biology. Inflammation Protocols, vol 225. Totowa (NJ): Humana Press; 2003. p. 378.

[82] Serhan CN, Gotlinger K, Hong S, et al. Anti-inflammatory actions of neuroprotectin D1/ protectin D1 and its natural stereoisomers: assignments of dihydroxy-containing docosatrienes. J Immunol 2006;176:1848–59.

[83] Capdevila JH, Wei S, Helvig C, et al. The highly stereoselective oxidation of polyunsaturated fatty acids by cytochrome P450BM-3. J Biol Chem 1996;271:22663–71.

[84] Arita M, Clish CB, Serhan CN. The contributions of aspirin and microbial oxygenase in the biosynthesis of anti-inflammatory resolvins: novel oxygenase products from omega-3 poly-unsaturated fatty acids. Biochem Biophys Res Commun 2005;338:149–57.

[85] Corey EJ, Shih C, Cashman JR. Docosahexaenoic acid is a strong inhibitor of prostaglandin but not leukotriene biosynthesis. Proc Natl Acad Sci U S A 1983;80:3581–4.

[86] Serhan CN, Oliw E. Unorthodox routes to prostanoid formation: new twists in cyclooxygenase-initiated pathways. J Clin Invest 2001;107:1481–9.

[87] Gronert K, Maheshwari N, Khan N, et al. A role for the mouse 12/15-lipoxygenase pathway in promoting epithelial wound healing and host defense. J Biol Chem 2005;280:15267–78.

[88] Hasturk H, Kantarci A, Ohira T, et al. RvE1 protects from local inflammation and osteoclast mediated bone destruction in periodontitis. FASEB J 2006;20:401–3.

[89] Duffield JS, Hong S, Vaidya V, et al. Omega-3 lipid mediators resolvin D and protectin D limit injury and acute renal failure following ischemia/reperfusion [abstract]. J Am Soc Nephrol 2005;16:17A.

[90] Ariel A, Li P-L, Wang W, Tang W-X, et al. The docosatriene protectin D1 is produced by T_H2 skewing and promotes human T cell apoptosis via lipid raft clustering. J Biol Chem 2005;280: 43079–86.

[91] Lukiw WJ, Cui JG, Marcheselli VL, et al. A role for docosahexaenoic acid-derived neuro-protectin D1 in neural cell survival and Alzheimer disease. J Clin Invest 2005;115:2774–83.

[92] Coffa G, Brash AR. A single active site residue directs oxygenation stereospecificity in lipoxygenases: stereocontrol is linked to the position of oxygenation. Proc Natl Acad Sci U S A 2004;101:15579–84.

[93] Hessler TG, Thomson MJ, Benscher D, et al. Association of a lipoxygenase locus, *Lpx-B1*, with variation in lipoxygenase activity in durum wheat seeds. Crop Science 2002;42:1695–700.

[94] Rådmark O. Arachidonate 5-lipoxygenase. Prostaglandins Other Lipid Mediat 2002;68–69: 211–34.

[95] Funk CD, Chen XS, Johnson EN, et al. Lipoxygenase genes and their targeted disruption. Prostaglandins Other Lipid Mediat 2002;68–69:303–12.

[96] Kuhn H, Thiele BJ. The diversity of the lipoxygenase family: many sequence data but little information on biological significance. FEBS Lett 1999;449:7–11.

[97] Furstenberger G, Marks F, Krieg P. Arachidonate 8(S)-lipoxygenase. Prostaglandins Other Lipid Mediat 2002;68–69:235–43.

[98] Vance RE, Hong S, Gronert K, Serhan CN, et al. The opportunistic pathogen *Pseudomonas aeruginosa* carries a novel secretable arachidonate 15-lipoxygenase. Proc Natl Acad Sci U S A 2004;101:2135–9.

[99] Hong S, Tjonahen E, Morgan EL, et al. Rainbow trout (*Oncorhynchus mykiss*) brain cells

biosynthesize novel docosahexaenoic acid-derived resolvins and protectins–mediator lipidomic analysis. Prostaglandins Other Lipid Mediat 2005;78:107–16.

[100] Rowley AF, Lloyd-Evans P, Barrow SE, et al. Lipoxin biosynthesis by trout macrophages involves the formation of epoxide intermediates. Biochemistry 1994;33:856–63.

[101] Majno G, Joris I. Cells, tissues, and disease: principles of general pathology. 2nd edition. New York: Oxford University Press; 2004.

[102] Samuelsson B, Dahlén SE, Lindgren JÅ, et al. Leukotrienes and lipoxins: structures, bio-synthesis, and biological effects. Science 1987;237:1171–6.

[103] Funk CD. Prostaglandins and leukotrienes: advances in eicosanoid biology. Science 2001;294: 1871–5.

[104] Capdevila JH, Falck JR, Dishman E, et al. Cytochrome P-450 arachidonate oxygenase. In: Murphy RC, Fitzpatrick FA, editors. Arachidonate related lipid mediators. vol. 187. San Diego (CA): Academic Press; 1990. p. 385–94.

[105] Node K, Huo Y, Ruan X, et al. Anti-inflammatory properties of cytochrome P450 epoxygenase-derived eicosanoids. Science 1999;285:1276–9.

[106] Rodriguez AR, Spur BW. First total synthesis of 7(*S*),16(*R*),17(*S*)-Resolvin D2, a potent anti-inflammatory lipid mediator. Tetrahedron Lett 2004;45:8717–20.

ELSEVIER
SAUNDERS

Anesthesiology Clin N Am
24 (2006) 365–379

ANESTHESIOLOGY
CLINICS OF
NORTH AMERICA

Pharmacologic Modulation of Operative Risk in Patients Who Have Cardiac Disease

Ashley M. Shilling, MD[a],*, Marcel E. Durieux, MD, PhD[a,b]

[a]Department of Anesthesia, University of Virginia Health System, Old Medical School, Room 4748, Charlottesville, VA 22908-0710, USA
[b]Department of Neurological Surgery, University of Virginia Medical Center, PO Box 800212, Charlottesville, VA, 22908, USA

One of the main goals of the practice of anesthesiology is to reduce risk in patients undergoing surgical operations. However, this is not easy to document. The specialty prides itself on major reductions in anesthesia-related mortality, but the validity of the supporting data has been questioned recently [1]. Attempts to reduce overall perioperative mortality (which hovers between 1% and 2%) may be even more difficult to study than reduced anesthetic risk, because so many more factors are involved. Because cardiovascular complications (in particular, cardiac death and myocardial infarction (MI) compose a major part of post-operative mortality, most studies have focused on this area. Some spectacular successes in perioperative interventions have been reported (eg, the long-term benefits of perioperative β-blockade), and these interventions have even become part of national protocols. However, as with touted reductions in anesthetic mortality, it pays to look carefully at the original data. Many of these studies have significant limitations, both in design and in patient population. Often the subjects were selected carefully and, therefore, data may not be applicable to the general population.

In this review, the authors discuss the most important studies of pharmacologic interventions aimed at preventing perioperative cardiovascular morbidity and mortality. A related topic, preventing neurocognitive dysfunction in patients undergoing cardiac surgery, is also discussed briefly.

---

* Corresponding author.
 E-mail address: abm5f@virginia.edu (A.M. Shilling).

0889-8537/06/$ – see front matter © 2006 Elsevier Inc. All rights reserved.
doi:10.1016/j.atc.2006.02.001

anesthesiology.theclinics.com

Cardiac outcome

β-Adrenergic blockade

The drug most likely to come to mind when discussing perioperative risk reduction is probably the β-adrenergic receptor antagonist. For years, it has been known that β-blockade reduces mortality after MI, is efficacious in the treatment of hypertension, and reduces the risk of ventricular arrhythmias. In the vascular surgery population, two studies have shown that perioperative β-blockade decreases the risk of perioperative MI and arrhythmias [2,3]. Attention became focused on this topic with a landmark trial by Mangano and colleagues [4] that indicated significant benefit of β-blockade in subjects who had cardiac risk factors and were undergoing noncardiac surgery. The investigators studied the use of perioperative atenolol continued until discharge, or seven days postoperatively, in 200 subjects who had either known coronary disease or greater than two risk factors for coronary artery disease, and were undergoing elective noncardiac surgery. For 2 years, they followed the 192 subjects who survived until hospital discharge. Overall mortality was reduced by 55% (P = .019) in the atenolol group and cardiovascular deaths were reduced by 65% (P = .033). In addition, the study demonstrated an increase in the length of time to first adverse event and in event-free survival in subjects given atenolol. The beneficial effects of atenolol were most evident during the first 6 to 8 months after surgery. These were highly encouraging data. However, this study has come under significant criticism [5]. Most importantly, the six in-hospital deaths were not included in the analysis; if these were included, the difference in death rates between the two groups would no longer be significant. In addition, the groups were not balanced as to risk factors: there were a greater number of diabetic patients in the group not receiving β-blockade.

In 1998, Wallace and colleagues [6] published a paper with data derived from Mangano's trial, evaluating perioperative myocardial ischemia as the primary outcome. They found that in β-blocked subjects, the postoperative incidence of ischemia was 50% lower in the first 48 hours (P = .008) and 40% lower during days 0 to 7 (P = .029). They also found that subjects with myocardial ischemia before, during, or after surgery were more likely to die within the next 2 years (P = .025), thus potentially explaining Mangano's finding that 7 days of treatment with atenolol could affect long-term morbidity.

Shortly after these studies, Poldermans and colleagues [7] published a randomized controlled trial looking at perioperative bisoprolol in subjects undergoing vascular surgery. Unlike the previous studies, every subject with one or more risk factors underwent dobutamine stress echocardiography, and only those with confirmed ischemia were included in the trial. These subjects were then randomized to receive either conventional therapy or bisoprolol for 30 days. The investigators found a decreased 30-day mortality (3.4% versus 17%) and a reduced incidence of nonfatal MI (0% versus 17%) in subjects treated with the β-blocker. A follow-up study by the same group [8] found similar long-term

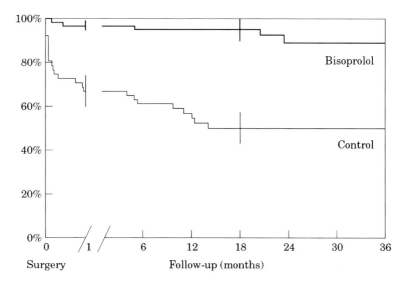

Fig. 1. Kaplan-Meier curves for cardiac death or MI during follow-up of 101 subjects who survived vascular surgery. Each plot represents the cumulative percentage of subjects remaining event-free.

benefits when following subjects from 11 months to a maximum of 30 months (median 22 months) after surgery (Fig. 1). The number of long-term cardiac events in the bisoprolol group was 12%, versus 32% in the control group (P=.025). Cardiac death occurred in 11% of the bisoprolol group, versus 20% in the standard care group, which was not significantly different (P=0.259). The end point of either cardiac death or nonfatal MI occurred in 12% of subjects receiving bisoprolol, versus 32% of standard care subjects (P=.025). The odds ratio for postoperative cardiac death or MI in high-risk subjects receiving bisoprolol therapy was 0.3 (90% confidence interval 0.11–0.83). Caution should be used, however, when interpreting this data because of the highly selected patient population included in the study: only subjects with documented myocardial ischemia were included. Polderman's trials, like Mangano's, have been criticized for the lack of blinding and for early termination because of the unexpectedly great risk reduction. In addition, the treatment effects have been considered "implausibly large" [5].

Building on studies by Poldermans, Kertai and colleagues [9] performed an observational study of the long-term outcome of subjects undergoing major vascular surgery, who survived 30 days postoperatively. Each of the 1351 subjects they screened who had one or more cardiovascular risk factors underwent dobutamine stress testing. The investigators followed 1286 subjects for a median of 23 months and, using multivariate analysis, found that β-blocker use was associated with a significantly reduced risk of late cardiac complications (adjusted hazard ratio [HR] 0.3; 95% confidence interval 0.2–0.6; P<.001). Using dobutamine stress echo, the investigators further risk-stratified the subjects and showed that even subjects without risk factors who took β-blockers showed an improved event-free survival (2.8% versus 0%). In subjects with one or two risk factors, the presence of ischemia on dobutamine stress echo increased the cardiac event rate from 3.9% to 9.8%, which was then reduced to 7.2% by the addition of peri-operative β-blockade. In subjects with three or more risk factors, but without ischemia on stress echo, β-blockade reduced the cardiac event rate from 15.1% to 9.5%. Finally, subjects with three risk factors and ischemia had a high event rate of 20.5%, even with β-blockade. The investigators concluded that perioperative β-blockade is useful in patients with two or fewer cardiac risk factors and documented ischemia, but may not be helpful in patients with three or more risk factors and documented ischemia. However, this was an observational study, not a randomized controlled trial, and as such has major inherent weaknesses.

The same caveat holds for a retrospective study by Taylor and Pagliarello [10], which looked at 236 subjects undergoing laparotomy. The investigators found, as expected, that postoperative cardiac events, including MI, ischemia, arrhythmia, congestive heart failure, and cardiac deaths, occurred more often in subjects who had documented coronary artery disease, but that β-blockers significantly de-creased the number. Subjects with only one risk factor or with no risk factors for coronary artery disease showed no benefit with the addition of β-blockade.

The largest study to date, a retrospective cohort study including data from 329 hospitals, looked at the use of perioperative β-blockers and their association with in-hospital mortality [11]. The study included 663,635 subjects undergoing major noncardiac surgery. Eighteen percent of these subjects met the investiga-tors' criteria for receiving perioperative β-blockade. The drug was administered on hospital days 1 or 2. Subjects receiving β-blockers after hospital day 2 were not considered part of the perioperative treatment group. Using propensity-score matching and multivariable logistic modeling, the investigators concluded that the use of perioperative β-blockade and risk of death varied with cardiac risk factors. The risk of in-hospital deaths was reduced among high-risk subjects who received perioperative β-blockers, and the number needed to treat to prevent one death was 33 in the highest-risk subjects. The use of perioperative β-blockers in subjects with low cardiac risk scores showed no benefit from β-blockers, and possible harm. Despite the large study size, limitations include the retrospective nature of the trial, the lack of randomization, and the restriction to in-hospital mortality.

In an attempt to sort out this confusing data, two meta-analyses have been performed on the use of β-blockers and cardiac events. The first, published in 2002 by Auerbach and Goldman [12], looked at five randomized controlled trials and the outcomes of myocardial ischemia, MI, cardiac death, and all-cause death. Four of the five studies found a statistical reduction in perioperative myocardial ischemia when β-blockers were given (Fig. 2). The study population of the group not reaching statistical difference underwent elective knee replacement. The numbers needed to treat to prevent cardiac or all-cause mortality ranged from 3.2 to 8.3. The greatest benefit was seen in subjects with the highest cardiac risk factors. The investigators noted the heterogeneity of the trials, and the lack of standardization and randomization of treatment protocols. Total enrollment in these trials was only 700 subjects, and, in essence, the current recommendations

Study or sub-category	β blocker (n/N)	Control (n/N)	Relative risk (99% CI)	Weight (%)	Relative risk (99% CI)
Jakobsen 1997[30]	1/18	0/18		5.29	3.00 (0.05 to 185.13)
Wallace[31]	3/99	5/101		16.38	0.61 (0.10 to 3.88)
Bayliff[32]	2/49	3/50		12.74	0.68 (0.07 to 6.74)
Poldermans[33]	2/59	18/53		16.27	0.10 (0.02 to 0.64)
Raby[34]	0/15	1/11		5.36	0.25 (0.00 to 14.93)
Zaugg[35]	0/43	3/20		5.98	0.07 (0.00 to 3.15)
Urban[36]	1/60	3/60		9.08	0.33 (0.02 to 6.29)
Yang[37]	19/246	22/250		28.90	0.88 (0.41 to 1.90)
Total	589	563		100.00	0.44 (0.16 to 1.24)

Total events: 28 (β blocker), 55 (control)

Test for heterogeneity: χ^2=12.07, df=7, P=0.10, I^2=42.0%

Test for overall effect: z=2.05, P=0.04

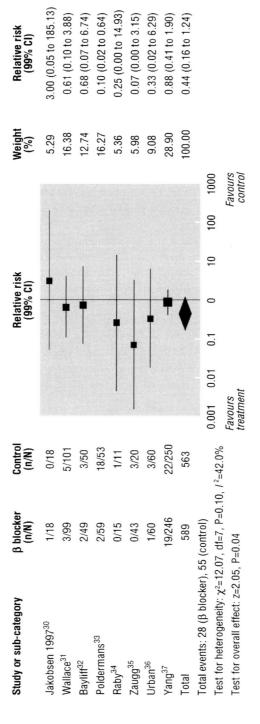

Fig. 2. Relative risk for major perioperative cardiovascular events (cardiac death, nonfatal MI, or nonfatal cardiac arrest).

are based on a total of 15 deaths and 18 nonfatal MIs (of which 11 deaths and 9 infarctions derive from a single trial) [7]. Nonetheless, the investigators concluded that the literature suggests beneficial effects of β-blockers on mortality and morbidity.

A recent meta-analysis and systematic review by Devereaux and colleagues [13] looked at a total of 22 randomized trials. Unlike the aforementioned analysis, this study looked at perioperative outcome within 30 days of surgery. The investigators found no statistically significant benefit for any of the individual outcomes and were only able to show a relative risk of 0.44 (95% confidence interval 0.20–0.97) for the combined outcomes of cardiovascular mortality, nonfatal MI, and nonfatal cardiac arrest. Furthermore, the study shows an increase in the incidence of bradycardia and hypotension requiring treatment when β-blockers were administered. Despite the suggestion that β-blockers may decrease the risk of major perioperative events, the investigators point out that these results are based on methodologically weak trials and a moderate number of major events.

Recently, American College of Cardiology and American Heart Association task force guidelines for noncardiac surgery have recommended perioperative β-blockade for vascular surgery patients with positive stress test (class I) and patients who have coronary artery disease, risk factors, or untreated hypertension (class IIA). These recommendations are still debated. To help with this debate, the authors are awaiting the results of the international Perioperative Ischemic Evaluations (POISE) trial, for which it is hoped that more than 10,000 subjects will be recruited.

Clonidine

A possible alternative to β-blockade might be the perioperative use of clonidine. Clonidine, a centrally acting α2 agonist, is used commonly to treat hypertension and decrease sympathetic discharge. It has the added benefits of providing anxiolysis, sedation, and analgesia, and decreasing anesthetic requirements [14]. Clonidine has also been shown to decrease shivering and oxygen consumption during anesthesia recovery [15]. During the last decade, clonidine has become a prevalent subject in the scientific literature and studies have demonstrated many perioperative benefits in patients being treated with this drug. Many of these studies are small, nonrandomized, or use surrogate rather than patient-important end points. Nonetheless, available data suggest that, in some settings, clonidine may reduce perioperative mortality, myocardial ischemia, and cortisol excretion, and may improve hemodynamics.

One of the earlier clonidine studies, by Dorman and colleagues [16], looked at the use of preoperative oral clonidine in 43 elective coronary artery bypass (CABG) subjects. They found the benefits of clonidine to include lower heart rates intra- and postoperatively, lower levels of serum epinephrine and norepinephrine, significantly less perioperative ST-segment depression, and a decreased need for sufentanil and enflurane. However, they also documented a decrease in perioperative cardiac output and an increased requirement for postoperative cardiac pacing. Despite these disadvantages, the investigators concluded that cloni-dine is safe in CABG subjects with normal cardiac conduction and ventricular function, and may reduce perioperative myocardial ischemia. Another study, by Myles and colleagues [17], examined the use of oral clonidine in 150 subjects undergoing elective CABG with a propofol anesthetic technique. Like Dorman and colleagues, they found a significant increase in bradycardia and postcardio-pulmonary bypass pacing requirements. Clonidine did not appear to prolong time to extubation or discharge from the ICU; in fact, the investigators actually demonstrated a decrease in time to extubation in subjects receiving clonidine. Unlike Dorman and colleagues, this group was unable to show a statistical dif-ference in perioperative myocardial ischemia, but the study did show favorable results in postoperative renal function and a reduction in urinary cortisol ex-cretion. The team also found significant improvement in the subjective health perception of the subjects postdischarge. Because sample sizes were relatively small and results varied with respect to subject and relevant outcome, the benefit of clonidine use in cardiac surgery patients must be considered unclear.

In addition to the use of perioperative clonidine in cardiac surgery, there have been several studies of clonidine use in noncardiac operations. Wallace and col-leagues [18] performed a double-blind trial of 190 subjects who had either known coronary disease, or risk factors for coronary disease, and were undergoing non-cardiac surgery. They showed a statistically significant decrease in perioperative myocardial ischemia and a decrease in 30-day and 2-year mortality in subjects administered a combination of perioperative oral and transdermal clonidine for 4 days (Fig. 3). They also found a decrease in serum epinephrine and norepi-

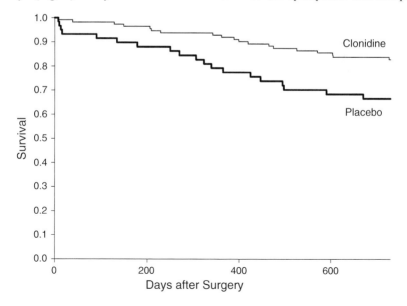

Fig. 3. Two-year postsurgery survival curves for subjects treated with clonidine (n=125) and a placebo (n=65). Clonidine statistically reduced the incidence of death.

nephrine levels in clonidine users. Ellis and colleagues [19] also studied the use of clonidine in subjects undergoing noncardiac surgery and found a reduction in intraoperative ischemia but no difference in postoperative myocardial ischemia. In another randomized trial, using 297 subjects undergoing noncardiac surgery, perioperative myocardial ischemia decreased from 39% to 24% in subjects randomized to clonidine [20]. There was no significant difference in hemodynamic patterns, MI, or mortality. A study by Hidalgo and colleagues [21] investigated preoperative oral clonidine in 61 subjects undergoing abdominal hysterectomy. They documented a statistically significant decrease in average heart rate perioperatively (68% of clonidine-receiving subjects had an average heart rate of less than 70, versus 21.9% in the placebo group).They also found that subjects receiving oral clonidine had less pain and anxiety after surgery. There was no statistical significance in hypotension or need for vasopressors.

In an attempt to understand better the perioperative benefits of clonidine, Nishina and colleagues [22] performed a meta-analysis of subjects receiving clonidine versus placebo. They included seven studies: five cardiac surgery and two noncardiac surgery. The investigators found the pooled odds ratio for the reduction of myocardial ischemia to be significant in the seven studies (0.49, 95% confidence interval 0.34–0.71). There was also a significant reduction in myocardial ischemia with clonidine use in the individual subgroups of cardiac and noncardiac surgery. While myocardial ischemia does not equate with mortality, it is known that even one episode of perioperative myocardial ischemia is associated with increased risk of 2-year mortality [23]. What is not known, however, is whether eliminating this episode of ischemia will decrease long-term mortality. The investigators noted several shortcomings of the study, including the difficulty in assessing ischemia in CABG subjects, and using the surrogate marker of ischemia. They calculated that more than 5000 subjects would need to be included in a trial to show differences in mortality and MI. Despite this, the investigators concluded that perioperative clonidine reduces ischemia episodes in patients who have known, or who are at risk for, coronary artery disease, without increasing the incidence of bradycardia.

At this point, there is a solid understanding of the mechanism of action of clonidine and its effects on the cardiovascular and autonomic systems. It seems intuitive that it could offer patient benefits of hemodynamic stability and a decreased stress response during surgery. Whether this would change perioperative morbidity or mortality is not as clear. Studies have demonstrated that clonidine reduces perioperative myocardial ischemia in patients undergoing CABG and those having noncardiac surgery, but myocardial ischemia is a surrogate end point. Only a single study has demonstrated a decrease in mortality in subjects receiving clonidine. This may be due to the low incidence of patient deaths in both cardiac and noncardiac surgery and the insufficient power of the existing trials. Based on available data, it seems prudent to use clonidine with caution in patients with conduction defects, although the incidence of significant bradycardia appears low and should not negatively affect the use of this potentially beneficial drug. It may be a particularly good drug choice in patients unable to take β-blockers. In addition to the reduction in myocardial ischemia, added benefits of clonidine include an anesthetic-sparing effect, an improvement in renal function, a decrease in pain and anxiety, and a decrease in serum catecholamine and urinary cortisol levels. Until further data are available, it is sensible to consider the use of perioperative clonidine in patients who have cardiovascular disease or those who have cardiac risk factors and are to undergo surgery.

Statins

While statins have been used for decades in both primary and secondary prevention of ischemic events, recent literature suggests that they may be useful drugs in the perioperative setting as well. These perioperative benefits probably are not a result of the cholesterol-lowering properties of the drugs. One of the earlier studies, the Cholesterol and Recurrent Events Trial (CARE) trial [24], followed 2245 subjects post-MI who were randomized to receive either pravastatin or a placebo. Subjects were started on pravastatin post-MI and then underwent coronary angioplasty, CAGB, or both, within the first 3 months of their MI. Not surprisingly, statin therapy resulted in a significant reduction in low-density lipoprotein levels. In addition, angioplasty subjects treated with statins had a 43% reduction in MI rate ($P=.009$), a 39% reduction in cardiovascular-related death ($P=.01$), and a 72% reduction in the incidence of stroke ($P=.006$). CABG subjects receiving statins had a 33% reduction in the incidence of cardiovascular death ($P=.034$). A similar trial, the Post-Coronary Artery Bypass Graft (Post-CABG) trial [25], looked at the effect of statin therapy started from 1 to 11 months post-CABG. Subjects receiving aggressive therapy with lovastatin not only had a 30% reduction in revascularization procedures ($P=.006$), but also a 24% reduction in the composite end points of cardiovascular death, death from any cause, stroke, and need for revascularization ($P=.001$). Both of these studies strongly suggest the importance of statin use in patients following CABG or stent procedures.

If postprocedure statins could statistically lower mortality and morbidity, then preoperative statins might be of even greater benefit. Many retrospective studies of cardiac surgery patients have been conducted to investigate this hypothesis. Dotani and coworkers [26] performed a retrospective cohort study of 323 subjects receiving statins before CABG, using the end points of death, MI, unstable angina, and arrhythmias. They found that preoperative statin therapy was associated with a significant reduction in the composite end points of death, unstable angina, and MI after CABG ($P=.02$), as well as with a decrease in the incidence of arrhythmias. Another retrospective cohort study, by Pan and colleagues [27], looked at preoperative statin therapy in 1663 subjects undergoing primary CABG. They found the 30-day all-cause mortality to be 50% lower in preoperative statin users (1.8% versus 3.75%; $P=.01$). The adjusted odds ratio for mortality in subjects receiving preoperative statins was 0.53 (95% confidence interval 0.28–0.99). No differences were observed in rates of postoperative MI, stroke, renal failure, or arrhythmias. In contrast to these findings, Ali and colleagues [28] retrospectively studied 1706 subjects who had unstable angina and were undergoing CABG or valve surgery. The end points chosen by this group included in-hospital mortality, intra- and postoperative need for intra-aortic balloon pump, perioperative MI, greater than 24 hours of postoperative mechanical ventilation, and stroke. After adjusting for covariables, the investigators did not find a statistical difference in mortality or any of the other end points in statin users. They concluded that preoperative statin use is not associated with a reduction in mortality or morbidity in patients who have unstable angina and are undergoing cardiac surgery.

The main caveat is that all these trials were retrospective. Unfortunately, no randomized, controlled, prospective trials are available in this population. Although these studies suggest that preoperative statin use may reduce morbidity and mortality in patients undergoing elective cardiac surgeries, more definitive data is required before any recommendations can be made. For patients who have unstable angina requiring urgent surgery, there seems to be little reason to consider statin use.

Many recent studies have looked at statin use in noncardiac surgery. Unfortunately, the majority of these are again retrospective reviews. Lindenauer and colleagues [29] performed a retrospective cohort of 780,591 subjects having intrathoracic, abdominal, or suprainguinal vascular surgery. They assigned each of the subjects a cardiac risk factor based on his or her medical history. The group found that subjects who were administered a statin within the first 2 hospital days had a statistical decrease in mortality (2.18% died, versus 3.15% in control subjects; $P<.001$). Using logistic regression, the risk of mortality was lower in treated subjects (odds ratio 0.62; 95% confidence interval 0.58–0.67). The number needed to treat to prevent one postoperative death was high: 85, ranging from 30 in subjects who had a high cardiac risk index to 186 in subjects who had no cardiac risks. The investigators concluded that perioperative statins decrease mortality, particularly in subjects at high risk for coronary disease.

Poldermans and colleagues' retrospective case-controlled study [30] looked at 2816 subjects undergoing vascular surgery and 160 subjects who died postoperatively during their hospital stay. They found that the risk of perioperative mortality was reduced 4.5 times in statin users, with an adjusted odds ratio of 0.22 (95% confidence interval 0.10–0.47). From this same study, the investigators concluded that statins demonstrate improved risk reduction over β-blockers, as the latter only provided a 2.3% reduction in cardiac mortality (adjusted odds ratio 0.43; 95% confidence interval 0.26–0.72). Further studies exist that support the use of statins in noncardiac surgery. Kertai and colleagues [31] performed a retrospective cohort study of 510 subjects and found a significant reduction in all-cause and cardiovascular mortality in statin users undergoing abdominal aortic aneurysm surgery. After adjusting for clinical risk factors and β-blocker use, the association between statins and reduced mortality was 0.4 (95% confidence interval 0.3–0.6; $P<.001$). They concluded that both all-cause and cardiovascular mortality are reduced significantly in statin users with a 2.5-fold reduction in all-cause mortality and a 3-fold reduction in cardiovascular mortality. In contrast, they found a 1.5-fold reduction in all-cause and cardiovascular mortality in subjects using β-blockers. Finally, a retrospective study by O'Neil-Callahan and colleagues [32] looking at statin use in noncardiac vascular surgery found that statin users had a decrease in the composite of death, MI, myocardial ischemia, congestive heart failure, and arrhythmias during hospitalization. After adjusting for age, heart function, and diabetes, they found the odds ratio to be 0.52 ($P=.001$) in statin users, versus nonusers. Their number needed to treat was 15 to avoid one cardiac complication.

One prospective study of statin use in noncardiac surgery has been reported to date. Durazzo and coworkers [33] performed a prospective, randomized, double-blind trial initiating atorvastatin 30 days before vascular surgery. The incidence of death, MI, unstable angina, and stroke was significantly less (8% versus 26%; $P=.031$) at 6 months in subjects treated with atorvastatin.

Taken together, the data suggest that preoperative statin therapy is associated with improved outcome in patients undergoing noncardiac surgery. All of the studies targeted a patient population undergoing vascular surgery, with the exception of Lindenauer's, which included abdominal and thoracic surgery. This patient population has a very high risk of cardiovascular morbidity and mortality and likely benefits more from statin use than do patients who have a lower incidence of cardiac disease.

Statins have multiple mechanisms of action. Aside from the well-known inhibition of 3-hydroxy-3-methylglutaryl-coenzyme A (HMG-CoA) reductase (the rate-limiting step in cholesterol synthesis), there is also a decrease in the synthesis of other isoprenoid mediators involved in the cholesterol pathway [34]. It is known that hypercholesterolemia impairs endothelial function and that lowering cholesterol can restore this function. Furthermore, statins increase nitric oxide bioavailability, which is important in vascular relaxation and inhibits platelet aggregation and smooth muscle proliferation [35]. Statins have other effects, including a decrease in inflammation and oxidative stress [36]. Clinically, they have been shown to decrease C-reactive protein and cytokines, improve fibrinolysis, and decrease thrombosis. Therefore, it seems feasible that improvements would be seen in patient outcome if statins were started even only days before surgical interventions, before any appreciable drop in cholesterol levels. Major side effects (rhabdomyolysis, myopathy, and hepatic dysfunction) are rare. Although the benefit of these drugs in high-risk patients is still to be established completely, the outlook is promising.

Cognitive dysfunction after cardiac surgery

In addition to cardiovascular complications, one major and troubling side effect of cardiac surgery is the high incidence of cognitive dysfunction. Up to 80% of patients undergoing cardiac procedures may suffer from this, and although symptoms tend to improve as time passes, 10% to 30% of patients still demonstrate cognitive decline 6 months after surgery [37–39]. Intraoperative cerebral microembolisms and hypoperfusion are the main postulated mechanisms. In both cases, an inflammatory response in the brain could aggravate the damage.

Recently, two pharmacologic approaches have been suggested to limit the degree of cognitive dysfunction after heart surgery: the serine protease inhibitor, aprotinin, and the local anesthetic, lidocaine.

Aprotinin

Aprotinin has been shown to decrease operative blood loss and the incidence of stroke in CABG patients [40]. A recent, randomized, controlled pilot study by Harmon and colleagues [41] shows promising data for use of aprotinin in preventing neurocognitive decline after CABG procedures. Although they enrolled only 36 subjects, the investigators concluded that fewer cognitive deficits were observed, both 4 days and 6 weeks postoperatively, in subjects receiving high-dose aprotinin during their cardiac procedures. The proposed mechanisms include anti-inflammatory effects and an as-yet-poorly understood neuroprotective effect. With this encouraging data, it is hoped a larger trial will follow.

Lidocaine

In addition to blocking Na channels, local anesthetics affect other signaling pathways, including those involved in the inflammatory response. As a result, they can significantly modulate inflammatory signaling [42]. This mechanism may explain in part why two trials have shown protective effects of lidocaine on neurocognitive outcome after cardiac procedures.

Mitchell and colleagues [43] studied 65 subjects undergoing left heart valve procedures. The subjects completed a battery of neuropsychological tests pre-operatively, as well as 10 days, 10 weeks, and 6 months postoperatively. Subjects received a 48-hour infusion of lidocaine (1 mg/min bolus, followed by 240 mg over the first hour and 120 mg over the second hour, followed by 60 mg/h thereafter), or a placebo, in a blind, randomized manner. Significantly, more placebo subjects had a deficit in at least one test at 10 days and 10 weeks, and in 6 out of 11 tests the lidocaine group showed superior sequential percentage change scores. The investigators concluded that lidocaine had a cerebral protective effect in this setting, at a level that was noticed by the subjects.

These data are supported by a study by Wang and colleagues [44] investigating 118 subjects undergoing CABG with cardiopulmonary bypass. These subjects were randomized to receive either lidocaine (1.5 mg/kg bolus followed by a 4 mg/min infusion during operation, and 4 mg/kg in the cardiopulmonary bypass priming solution) or a placebo. Neuropsychological tests were administered before, and 9 days after, surgery. The proportion of subjects showing post-operative cognitive dysfunction was significantly reduced in the lidocaine group, compared with the placebo group.

Neither of these two studies is completely conclusive. However, they both have the strengths of being randomized, blind and placebo controlled, and their similar outcomes suggest that a large-scale trial of this safe and inexpensive approach might well be warranted.

Summary

Cardiac complications continue to compose a major proportion of serious postoperative morbidity and mortality, and it is appropriate, therefore, that this area has received a lot of attention in the search for pharmacologic modulation of surgical outcomes. Despite numerous studies, conclusive data does not exist, making it difficult to recommend a course of action. β-blockade has not only made it into national protocols, but is even considered as a quality assessment measure. However, the data are not quite as conclusive as it may sometimes appear. There have been few studies, with a small number of negative outcomes, and, at times, significant methodological concerns. The positive outcomes of meta-analyses rest essentially on a single trial [7] in a highly selected patient population. Although use of β-blockers in patients who have documented coronary artery disease and are undergoing major vascular procedures appears supported, it is premature to recommend β-blockade for all patients with cardiac risk. Because these drugs are not without risks, it might be advisable to be restrained in their use until the results of the large-scale randomized POISE trial are available.

For clonidine and statins, the data are even more tenuous, and largely based on retrospective reviews (with the exception of postprocedure use of statins, which is well supported). Here again, the results of large-scale prospective trials must become available before recommendations can be made.

Finally, promising data indicate that it might be possible to modulate by pharmacologic means the neurocognitive decline that is frequently associated with cardiac surgery, and which is often considered by patients to be the most troublesome complication of the intervention.

References

[1] Lagasse RS. Anesthesia safety: model or myth? A review of the published literature and analysis of current original data [comment]. Anesthesiology 2002;97(6):1609–17.
[2] Pasternack PF, Imparato AM, Baumann FG, et al. The hemodynamics of beta-blockade in patients undergoing abdominal aortic aneurysm repair. Circulation 1987;76(3 Pt 2):III1–7.
[3] Yeager RA, Moneta GL, Edwards JM, et al. Reducing perioperative myocardial infarction following vascular surgery. The potential role of beta-blockade. Arch Surg 1995;130(8):869–72 [discussion: 872–3].
[4] Mangano DT, Layug EL, Wallace A, et al. Effect of atenolol on mortality and cardiovascular morbidity after noncardiac surgery. Multicenter Study of Perioperative Ischemia Research Group [comment]. N Engl J Med 1996;335(23):1713–20 [erratum: N Engl J Med 1997;336(14):1039].

[5] Devereaux PJ, Leslie K, Yang H. The effect of perioperative beta-blockers on patients undergoing noncardiac surgery—is the answer in? [comment]. Can J Anaesth 2004;51(8):749–55.
[6] Wallace A, Layug B, Tateo I, et al. Prophylactic atenolol reduces postoperative myocardial ischemia. McSPI Research Group [comment]. Anesthesiology 1998;88(1):7–17.
[7] Poldermans D, Boersma E, Bax JJ, et al. The effect of bisoprolol on perioperative mortality and myocardial infarction in high-risk patients undergoing vascular surgery. Dutch Echocardiographic Cardiac Risk Evaluation Applying Stress Echocardiography Study Group [comment]. N Engl J Med 1999;341(24):1789–94.
[8] Poldermans D, Boersma E, Bax JJ, et al. Bisoprolol reduces cardiac death and myocardial infarction in high-risk patients as long as 2 years after successful major vascular surgery [comment]. Eur Heart J 2001;22(15):1353–8.
[9] Kertai MD, Boersma E, Bax JJ, et al. Optimizing long-term cardiac management after major vascular surgery: Role of beta-blocker therapy, clinical characteristics, and dobutamine stress echocardiography to optimize long-term cardiac management after major vascular surgery. Arch Intern Med 2003;163(18):2230–5.
[10] Taylor RC, Pagliarello G. Prophylactic beta-blockade to prevent myocardial infarction perioperatively in high-risk patients who undergo general surgical procedures. Can J Surg 2003; 46(3):216–22.
[11] Lindenauer PK, Pekow P, Wang K, et al. Perioperative beta-blocker therapy and mortality after major noncardiac surgery [comment]. N Engl J Med 2005;353(4):349–61.
[12] Auerbach AD, Goldman L. beta-Blockers and reduction of cardiac events in noncardiac surgery: scientific review [comment]. JAMA 2002;287(11):1435–44.
[13] Devereaux PJ, Beattie WS, Choi PT, et al. How strong is the evidence for the use of perioperative beta blockers in non-cardiac surgery? Systematic review and meta-analysis of randomised controlled trials. BMJ 2005;331(7512):313–21.
[14] Flacke JW, Bloor BC, Flacke WE, et al. Reduced narcotic requirement by clonidine with improved hemodynamic and adrenergic stability in patients undergoing coronary bypass surgery. Anesthesiology 1987;67(1):11–9.
[15] Quintin L, Bouilloc X, Butin E, et al. Clonidine for major vascular surgery in hypertensive patients: a double-blind, controlled, randomized study. Anesth Analg 1996;83(4):687–95.
[16] Dorman BH, Zucker JR, Verrier ED, et al. Clonidine improves perioperative myocardial ischemia, reduces anesthetic requirement, and alters hemodynamic parameters in patients undergoing coronary artery bypass surgery [comment]. J Cardiothorac Vasc Anesth 1993;7(4):386–95.
[17] Myles PS, Hunt JO, Holdgaard HO, et al. Clonidine and cardiac surgery: haemodynamic and metabolic effects, myocardial ischaemia and recovery. Anaesth Intensive Care 1999;27(2):137–47.
[18] Wallace AW, Galindez D, Salahieh A, et al. Effect of clonidine on cardiovascular morbidity and mortality after noncardiac surgery. Anesthesiology 2004;101(2):284–93.
[19] Ellis JE, Drijvers G, Pedlow S, et al. Premedication with oral and transdermal clonidine provides safe and efficacious postoperative sympatholysis. Anesth Analg 1994;79(6):1133–40.
[20] Stuhmeier KD, Mainzer B, Cierpka J, et al. Small, oral dose of clonidine reduces the incidence of intraoperative myocardial ischemia in patients having vascular surgery. Anesthesiology 1996; 85(4):706–12.
[21] Hidalgo MP, Auzani JA, Rumpel LC, et al. The clinical effect of small oral clonidine doses on perioperative outcomes in patients undergoing abdominal hysterectomy. Anesth Analg 2005; 100(3):795–802.
[22] Nishina K, Mikawa K, Uesugi T, et al. Efficacy of clonidine for prevention of perioperative myocardial ischemia: a critical appraisal and meta-analysis of the literature. Anesthesiology 2002;96(2):323–9.
[23] Mangano DT, Browner WS, Hollenberg M, et al. Long-term cardiac prognosis following noncardiac surgery. The Study of Perioperative Ischemia Research Group [comment]. JAMA 1992;268(2):233–9.
[24] Sacks FM, Pfeffer MA, Moye LA, et al. The effect of pravastatin on coronary events after myocardial infarction in patients with average cholesterol levels. Cholesterol and Recurrent Events Trial investigators [comment]. N Engl J Med 1996;335(14):1001–9.

[25] The Post-CABG Trial Investigators. The effect of aggressive lowering of low-density lipoprotein levels and anticoagulation on obstructive changes in saphenous vein coronary-artery bypass grafts. N Engl J Med 1997;336:153–62.
[26] Dotani MI, Elnicki DM, Jain AC, et al. Effect of preoperative statin therapy and cardiac outcomes after coronary artery bypass grafting. Am J Cardiol 2000;86(10):1128–30.
[27] Pan W, Pintar T, Anton J, et al. Statins are associated with a reduced incidence of perioperative mortality after coronary artery bypass graft surgery. Circulation 2004;110(Suppl 1):II45–9.
[28] Ali IS, Buth KJ. Preoperative statin use and in-hospital outcomes following heart surgery in patients with unstable angina. Eur J Cardiothorac Surg 2005;27(6):1051–6.
[29] Lindenauer PK, Pekow P, Wang K, et al. Lipid-lowering therapy and in-hospital mortality following major noncardiac surgery. JAMA 2004;291(17):2092–9.
[30] Poldermans D, Bax JJ, Kertai MD, et al. Statins are associated with a reduced incidence of perioperative mortality in patients undergoing major noncardiac vascular surgery [comment]. Circulation 2003;107(14):1848–51.
[31] Kertai MD, Boersma E, Westerhout CM, et al. Association between long-term statin use and mortality after successful abdominal aortic aneurysm surgery. Am J Med 2004;116(2):96–103.
[32] O'Neil-Callahan K, Katsimaglis G, Tepper MR, et al. Statins decrease perioperative cardiac complications in patients undergoing noncardiac vascular surgery: the Statins for Risk Reduction in Surgery (StaRRS) study. J Am Coll Cardiol 2005;45(3):336–42.
[33] Durazzo AE, Machado FS, Ikeoka DT, et al. Reduction in cardiovascular events after vascular surgery with atorvastatin: a randomized trial [comment]. J Vasc Surg 2004;39(5):967–75 [discussion: 975–6].
[34] Lazar HL. Role of statin therapy in the coronary bypass patient. Ann Thorac Surg 2004;78(2):730–40.
[35] Laufs U, La Fata V, Plutzky J, et al. Upregulation of endothelial nitric oxide synthase by HMG CoA reductase inhibitors. Circulation 1998;97(12):1129–35.
[36] Takemoto M, Liao JK. Pleiotropic effects of 3-hydroxy-3-methylglutaryl coenzyme a reductase inhibitors. Arterioscler Thromb Vasc Biol 2001;21(11):1712–9.
[37] Sotaniemi KA, Mononen H, Hokkanen TE. Long-term cerebral outcome after open-heart surgery. A five-year neuropsychological follow-up study. Stroke 1986;17(3):410–6.
[38] Selnes OA, Goldsborough MA, Borowicz LM, et al. Neurobehavioural sequelae of cardiopulmonary bypass. Lancet 1999;353(9164):1601–6.
[39] Newman MF, Kirchner JL, Phillips-Bute B, et al. Longitudinal assessment of neurocognitive function after coronary-artery bypass surgery [comment]. N Engl J Med 2001;344(6):395–402 [erratum: N Engl J Med 2001;344(24):1876].
[40] Murkin JM. Attenuation of neurologic injury during cardiac surgery. Ann Thorac Surg 2001;72(5):S1838–44.
[41] Harmon DC, Ghori KG, Eustace NP, et al. Aprotinin decreases the incidence of cognitive deficit following CABG and cardiopulmonary bypass: a pilot randomized controlled study [comment]. Can J Anaesth 2004;51(10):1002–9.
[42] Hollmann MW, Durieux ME. Local anesthetics and the inflammatory response: a new therapeutic indication? Anesthesiology 2000;93(3):858–75.
[43] Mitchell SJ, Pellett O, Gorman DF. Cerebral protection by lidocaine during cardiac operations. Ann Thorac Surg 1999;67(4):1117–24.
[44] Wang D, Wu X, Li J, et al. The effect of lidocaine on early postoperative cognitive dysfunction after coronary artery bypass surgery [comment]. Anesth Analg 2002;95(5):1134–41.

ELSEVIER
SAUNDERS

Anesthesiology Clin N Am
24 (2006) 381–405

ANESTHESIOLOGY
CLINICS OF
NORTH AMERICA

Interactions of Volatile Anesthetics with Neurodegenerative-Disease-Associated Proteins

Anna Carnini, PhD, Maryellen Fazen Eckenhoff, PhD,
Roderic G. Eckenhoff, MD*

*Department of Anesthesiology and Critical Care, University of Pennsylvania Health Systems,
305 John Morgan Building, 3620 Hamilton Walk, Philadelphia, PA 19104, USA*

The increased life expectancy of humans is associated with an increased prevalence of age-related disorders, including various disorders of cognition. The most common of such disorders is Alzheimer's disease, which is estimated to afflict 30 million people worldwide. According to predictions, 13 million people in the United States will have Alzheimer's disease in 2050. That's up from 4.5 million people in 2000 [1]. This alarming trend is a product of increasing life expectancy, which is now approaching 80 years of age, and the large bolus of individuals from the post-World War II baby boom now approaching retirement. The current medical and long-term care infrastructure is unprepared for the impending load, and the implications to our economy and culture cannot be understated [2].

Recently, there has been considerable emphasis on defining the risk factors and mechanisms of these cognitive disorders with the goal of reducing the prevalence. While a cure is desirable, the multifactorial nature of the various disorders has made this unlikely. Emphasis has shifted to therapy that can delay symptom onset and the identification of environmental factors that contribute to the pathogenesis of these neurodegenerative diseases. Our modern technological society unavoidably exposes individuals to stresses, conditions, chemicals, and pathogens that can contribute to the progression of many disorders, including dementias. Avoidance strategies receive less attention than novel therapeutics. However, such strategies may be more effective in many cases in reducing the

This work was supported by Grant No.AG23540 from the National Institute on Aging.

* Corresponding author.

E-mail address: roderic.eckenhoff@uphs.upenn.edu (R.G. Eckenhoff).

anesthesiology.theclinics.com

onset of dementia. For example, it is fairly well established that certain pesticides contribute to Parkinson's disease in workers and farmers so exposed [3]. Another example is the solvent trichloroethylene, which is used extensively in the electronics industry. Chronic exposure to trichloroethylene is now recognized as responsible for a wide spectrum of central nervous system effects, including confusion, problems with memory, and sensory disability [4]. Trichloroethylene was also a widely used volatile anesthetic in the middle of the twentieth century, and it is probable that millions of people were exposed to this chemical at much higher concentrations than current industrial limits. Do these patients today have residual central nervous system effects, or is there a greater incidence of Alzheimer's disease in this population? The data required to answer this question are not yet available, but a larger and more sobering question is whether currently used volatile anesthetics share this property. Well over 30 million people receive general anesthesia for surgical and other painful procedures every year in the United States alone and it is now recognized that cognitive decline after surgery occurs, especially in the elderly [5–9]. The overwhelming majority of general anesthetics include administration of a volatile halogenated hydrocarbon, not unlike trichloroethylene (Fig. 1). While the overall immediate risk appears to be very low, and the benefits enormous, the question of whether anesthetics may have serious side effects, specifically with respect to central nervous system function in the elderly, is now being asked by several investigators. Is it only a coincidence that Dr. Alois Alzheimer described his first patient in 1907, only a few decades after the introduction of volatile general anesthesia in 1846? In this review, the authors will address the possibility that volatile anesthetics specifically enhance the neurodegenerative disorders through a common biophysical mechanism. Evidence in support of this possibility is currently weak and indirect. This means that alarm or a change in practice is not currently justified. Nevertheless, the growing tsunami of dementia requires that clinician scientists leave no stone

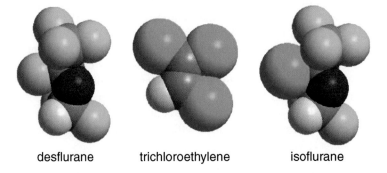

desflurane   trichloroethylene   isoflurane

Fig. 1. Three inhalational anesthetic molecules. Trichloroethylene, which is no longer used clinically, has been linked to chronic central nervous system disturbances. Isoflurane is currently the most commonly used inhalational anesthetic. Desflurane is another commonly used inhalational anesthetic. Note the similar size, shape, halogenation, and lack of charged atoms. Carbon=gray; oxygen=red; hydrogen=white; fluorine=light green; chlorine=dark green.

Table 1
Some neurodegenerative diseases

Disease	Regions of the brain affected	Pathological hallmarks	Protein deposited
Alzheimer's disease	Cortex, hippocampus, basal forebrain, brain stem	Neuritic plaques and neurofibrillary tangles	Amyloid β_{40}, amyloid β_{42}, tau
Parkinson's disease	Substantia nigra, cortex, locus ceruleus	Lewy bodies	α-Synuclein
Polyglutamine repeat diseases (Huntington's disease, spinobulbar muscular atrophy disease, and spinocerebellar ataxia)	Huntington's disease: striatum, basal ganglia, cortex, as well as other regions	Ubiquinated, neuronal nuclear inclusions	Huntingtin disease, atrophin-1, ataxins
Prion diseases (scrapie, mad cow, and Creutzfeldt-Jakob diseases)	Cortex, thalamus, brain stem, cerebellum, and other regions	Accumulation of protease-resistant prion protein aggregates, spongiform degeneration	Prion proteins, PrP

unturned in the quest to mitigate damage. Before discussing the potential anesthetic interactions, it is necessary to have a basic understanding of the features and pathogenesis of these disorders (Table 1).

Neurodegenerative diseases

Alzheimer's disease

Alzheimer's disease is a progressive disorder of cognition and memory. The principle risk factor is age, although several genetic predispositions have been identified [10,11]. Early descriptions of the brain pathology associated with Alzheimer's disease noted dense lesions, called plaque, in the brain parenchyma (Fig. 2). A large fraction of this plaque was found to be a single protein, amyloid beta (β). The term "amyloid" refers to the general appearance on light microscopy, and "beta" refers to the predominant form of secondary structure found in this proteinaceous material. Electron microscopy established this material's fibrillar nature, which is now well known [12]. Current work is attempting to establish the exact structure and the nature of the assembly.

The amyloid β peptide itself is a cleavage product from a large type I transmembrane protein called amyloid precursor protein (APP) (Fig. 3). The primary role of APP is not yet clear, but it is expressed by most cells of the central nervous system, and its deletion has been found to cause cognitive impairments and disruptions in hippocampal neuronal circuitry [13–15], suggesting that APP is important for normal brain development and function. The presenilins are

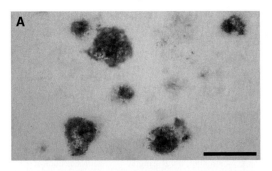

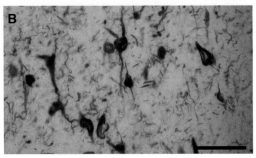

Fig. 2. Plaques and tangles in a human brain affected by Alzheimer's disease. (*A*) Example of extracellular plaque visualized with immunofluorescence using anti-amyloid β_{42} antibody (scale bar=125 μm). (*B*) Example of the intracellular neurofibrillary tangles visualized with anti-paired-helical-filiments-1 antibody (scale bar=62.5 μm). (*From* LaFerla FM, Oddo S. Alzheimer's disease: Abeta, tau and synaptic dysfunction. Trends Mol Med 2005;11(4):170.)

integral membrane proteins that regulate the β- and γ-secretase cleavages of APP releasing the amyloid β_{1-40} and amyloid β_{42} fragments. Soluble amyloid β_{40} and amyloid β_{1-42} are normally cleared from the cells and extracellular space, with no detrimental effects, through processes still not well understood. However, when the concentration of these hydrophobic peptides exceed their solubility, a self-assembly cascade begins, resulting ultimately in the amyloid fibril. The key role of amyloid β is formalized in the amyloid cascade hypothesis, which states that amyloid β is the most proximal trigger for Alzheimer's disease [16]. This hypothesis has been recently expanded to accommodate new information on the complexity of the cascade, and on the relative cytotoxicity. For example, the large fibrillar form of amyloid β was initially considered the toxic species, but now attention has shifted to earlier forms in the amyloid cascade, because plaque or fibril load does not correlate well with the degree of neurodegeneration [17] or central nervous system impairment. En route to fibril formation, amyloid β monomers can assemble into small aggregates of perhaps 5 to 20 monomers, such as protofibrils and small oligomers, which are still diffusible [18]. There is increasing experimental evidence that these small soluble intermediates are the main toxic form of the amyloid β peptide and are the basis of neurodegeneration in Alzheimer's disease [18–21]. This understanding has forced a reevaluation of

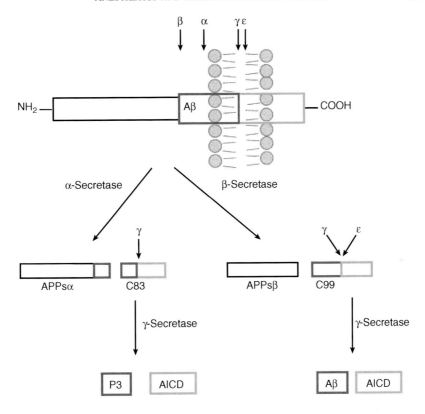

Fig. 3. The production of amyloid β peptide from APP. APP is a type 1 transmembrane protein (one pass through the membrane) cleaved by several proteases to produce a variety of products. Two particular cleavage sites, under the control of presenilin-1 and β-secretase, produce amyloid β_{40} or amyloid β_{42}, the two most common peptides in plaque. Certain mutations in APP increase the β site cleavages, resulting in a higher concentration of amyloid β peptide. Aβ, amyloid β; AICD, amyloid β precursor protein intracellular domain; COOH, carboxyl group; NH2, amino group. (*From* LaFerla FM, Oddo S. Alzheimer's disease: Abeta, tau and synaptic dysfunction. Trends Mol Med 2005;11(4):171.)

the extracellular plaque, which is now considered to be a less toxic or nontoxic sequestered form of the misfolded material [17]. In support of this idea is the finding that clearance and chaperonin proteins, such as ubiquitin and heat shock proteins, are found in plaque [22], along with amyloid β_{40} and amyloid β_{42}.

Discovering the toxic species in the amyloid cascade is central to developing appropriate therapeutics. For example, small molecules designed to inhibit plaque formation may increase the concentration of their precursor oligomers in the process, which is now predicted to enhance neurodegeneration. Recent effort is directed at reducing the early oligomerization events by decreasing the concentration of amyloid β peptide, increasing its solubility by prevention of amyloid β aggregation, or enhancing degradation [23–26]. Of interest are recent amyloid β immunotherapy studies. Active immunization by the administration of aggregated or soluble amyloid β peptides has been shown to inhibit amyloid β deposition in several transgenic mouse models [27–30] and in a nonhuman primate [31]. Passive immunization with polyclonal or monoclonal amyloid β antibodies can also prevent amyloid β plaques in transgenic mice [32–35]. Recently, it has been shown that a single intrahippocampal injection of an amyloid β antibody in 12-month-old triple-transgenic mice reduced extracellular amyloid β plaques and intracellular amyloid β accumulation, and also reduced early tau pathology [34]. Research has also shown that the intraneuronal amyloid β may be a source of the extracellular amyloid β plaques [36]. In addition to salutary effects on the pathology, both active and passive amyloid β immunization have been shown to prevent, lessen, or reverse cognitive deficits in transgenic mice [29,30,37,38], demonstrating the biological significance of the histology results. Human trials with the aggregated amyloid $β_{42}$ peptide were not as successful. Several patients developed meningoencephalitis in the phase II study, and the trials were terminated early [39,40]. There are also a number of in vitro studies using small-molecule amyloid β aggregation inhibitors [41–43]. Finally, many other therapies aimed more generically at apoptosis, inflammation, and signaling are underway. A description of these is beyond the scope of this review, but clearly not irrelevant to the issue of potential anesthetic effects.

In addition to deposits of fibrillar amyloid β peptides, human brain pathology of Alzheimer's disease is characterized by the presence of filamentous tau intracellular inclusions, termed neurofibrillary tangles (see Fig. 2) [44,45]. Neurofibrillary tangles consist of fibrils of an excessively phosphorylated form of the protein tau, whose function in the cell is to maintain the structural integrity of microtubules. Normally, tau is a soluble protein that promotes the assembly and stabilization of microtubules. Tau phosphorylation and oligomerization into fibrils remove tau from the tubulin oligomer (microtubule), which then becomes unstable and dissociates into soluble tubulin. The consequences to neuronal function, axonal transport, and synaptic function are predictably detrimental. Neurofibrillary tangles are found in the neurons of patients with Alzheimer's disease and other neurodegenerative disorders that in the absence of extracellular amyloid β deposits are known as tauopathies. These disorders include Alzheimer's disease, frontal temporal dementia with Parkinson's linked to chromosome 17, Pick's disease, progressive supranuclear palsy, and corticobasal degeneration [46]. While it is thought that tau pathology lies downstream of amyloid β pathology in the neurodegenerative cascade, it may prove important in the development of the clinical syndrome of Alzheimer's disease. Thus, a combination of these two protein oligomerization events appears to cooperatively produce neurodegeneration and, ultimately, cognitive symptoms.

Parkinson's disease

In contrast to Alzheimer's disease, which is the most common cognitive disorder, Parkinson's disease is the most common of the neurodegenerative movement disorders. Like Alzheimer's disease, the incidence of Parkinson's disease increases with age. According to estimates, the percentage of the population afflicted with Parkinson's disease increases from 1% at age 65, to 5% by age 85 [47]. Clinically, this disease is characterized by tremor, difficulty in maintaining balance, and overall slowness of movement. The pathological hallmark of this neurodegenerative disorder is the loss of dopaminergic neurons from the substantia nigra, and the formation of fibrillar intracellular inclusions called Lewy bodies [48]. The principal component of the Lewy body is α-synuclein, a small peptide belonging to the larger family of synuclein proteins. These proteins are abundant in the brain, particularly in nerve terminals. Although there are at least three types of human synuclein—α, β and γ—Lewy bodies contain exclusively α-synuclein. Mutations in the α-synuclein gene have been identified in familial Parkinson's disease and other neurological disorders [49–51]. A whole class of diseases has been named α-synucleinopathies and include Parkinson's disease, Lewy body disease, and multiple system atrophy [49]. Similar to amyloid β, the α-synuclein monomer is largely unstructured, oligomerizes to form fibrils, and is the current focus for therapeutics. Recent studies have found that amyloid β stimulates tau and α-synuclein pathology [52,53] and that α-synuclein stimulates tau pathology [54–56].

Polyglutamine repeat diseases

Polyglutamine (polyQ) diseases are due to alterations in protein conformations [57]. This group includes at least nine neurodegenerative diseases, such as Huntington's disease, spinobulbar muscular atrophy disease, dentatorubro-pallidolysian atrophy, and six forms of spinocerebellar ataxias. PolyQ disease is caused by CAG trinucleotide repeat expansion in the coding regions of disease-related genes, which produces, when translated, an expanded glutamine domain. The proteins containing this expanded glutamine domain form intracellular insoluble aggregates, maturing to fibrils rich in β sheet character, which are associated with neuronal degeneration.

Prion disorders

Prion protein diseases encompass a recently recognized and heterogeneous group of infectious diseases, including scrapie, which affects sheep and goats; bovine spongiform encephalopathy, which is commonly known as mad cow disease and which affects cattle; chronic wasting disease, which affects deer and elk; and Creutzfeldt-Jakob disease and kuru, which affect humans [58,59]. Clinically they manifest as slowly progressive dementia, which includes psychiatric disturbances, myoclonus, insomnia, and ataxia. Pathological manifestations include the accumulation of protease-resistant prion protein aggregates in affected brain regions [60]. The prion protein normally exists as a stable and structured conformer, whose physiological function is not clear. When misfolded, however, these proteins have the capacity to "catalytically" misfold native-state proteins, initiating an oligomerization cascade and forming toxic species. This self-catalytic property gives these proteins an infectious character, explaining why these diseases were initially thought to be caused by viruses. This accumulation of misfolded material may take years to evolve, producing a gradual spongiform encephalopathy. But again, the essential biophysical features of misfolding and aggregation are a highly conserved feature of most neurodegenerative disorders.

A common biophysical mechanism of neurodegeneration

Although a universal mechanism for the neurodegenerative diseases described above remains elusive, it is now apparent that a common feature in these diseases is the aggregation of misfolded or unfolded proteins [19,61,62] into a variety of oligomers, most of which go on to form fibrils. As indicated above, these aggregates have been identified in almost all forms of progressive neurodegenerative disease [63,64]. Are there unifying features of these assemblies that can form the basis of therapeutics, or perhaps provide hints as to the pathogenesis? A common secondary structural feature of these aggregates is a criss-cross pattern, known as a cross-β-sheet secondary structure [65] (Fig. 4). Many proteins, perhaps even all proteins, can be made to assume this structure and to

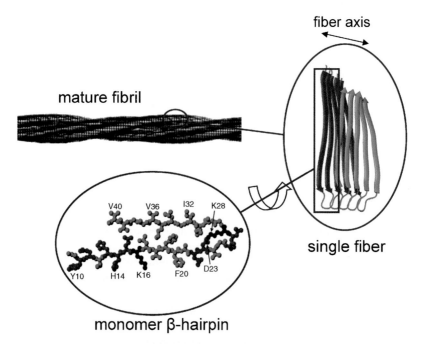

Fig. 4. Consensus structure of a cross-β protein fibril, in this case amyloid β_{40}. The β strands are oriented perpendicular to the long axis of the fibril, and each fibril is twisted with about three others to form the mature fibril. (*Adapted from* Stromer T, Serpell LC. Structure and morphology of the Alzheimer's amyloid fibril. Microsc Res Tech 2005;67(3–4):215; and Petkova AT, Ishii Y, Balbach JJ, et al. A structural model for Alzheimer's beta-amyloid fibrils based on experimental constraints from solid state NMR. Proc Natl Acad Sci USA 2002;99(26):16746, with permission.

form fibrils under the right conditions, especially those conditions that cause unfolding. This form of a normally nontoxic protein is often toxic. Might a common biophysical mechanism initiate neurodegeneration? The proteins discussed above, such as amyloid β and α-synuclein, may cause disease because they are already unfolded under biological conditions. This introduces the second unifying feature: The disease-associated protein monomers are unstable, essentially without structure. This feature contributes to the oligomerization through an ability of the monomer to continuously sample conformations suitable for binding with another monomer like itself. In turn, these unitary biophysical features suggest the intriguing possibility of a unified biophysical approach to therapeutics. Of course, this works both ways. The likelihood exists that other biophysical influences might enhance the progression of disease. Such a possibility opens the door for the consideration of environmental factors affecting the patient, including exposure to exogenous chemicals, such as anesthetics.

Biophysical basis for interactions of volatile anesthetics with neurodegenerative-disease-associated proteins

How might volatile anesthetics enhance the progression of neurodegenerative diseases? Aside from the features introduced above, such as β structure and instability, the key feature relevant to anesthetics is hydrophobicity. The hydrophobic effect provides the initial driving force bringing the oligomer together. As monomers assemble as a result of the hydrophobic force, small oligomers adjust their conformation to maximize hydrogen bonding, in which hydrophobic interactions continue to play a major role [66], resulting ultimately in the characteristic cross-β structure. The resulting small molecular aggregates further assemble and adjust conformation to produce fibrils, an enormous, highly organized and essentially irreversible oligomer. These assemblies can be cooperatively stabilized by other molecules, ions, and proteins in the cell. Interactions between these proteins are common, as noted above. Further, there are permissive interactions between tau and amyloid β that are also poorly understood [67]. In the end, all of these interactions produce exceptionally stable fibrils, although at least in the case of the amyloid β, the immunotherapy studies (see above) have suggested that reversibility can occur in vivo [38].

The authors have proposed that inhaled anesthetics accelerate protein oligomerization because of their unique physical properties and because such anesthetics are present in relatively high concentration (ie, high micromolar levels) during a typical general anesthetic. The inhaled anesthetics are made up of small, relatively inert hydrophobic molecules that bind preferentially in internal protein cavities [68,69]. These compounds can enhance protein-protein interactions, and therefore oligomer formation, in two ways. First, as the authors have reported, these gases favor protein intermediates with enlarged cavities, and thus cause destabilization and enhance disorder in some proteins [70,71]. As also stated, this promotes the entropic freedom to sample conformations capable of self-

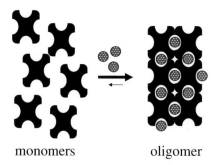

monomers   oligomer

Fig. 5. Many protein-protein surfaces contain packing defects (also called uncomplemented pockets), which form a suitable anesthetic binding site only in the oligomer. The presence of an anesthetic (dotted ovals) stabilizes the complex, shifting the equilibrium in that direction, effectively decreasing the concentration of monomer necessary to initiate oligomer formation.

recognition and aggregation. Second, hydrophobic cavities of suitable volume for anesthetic binding are often formed at protein-protein interfaces [72]. Because cavity formation is energetically unfavorable, the protein-protein interaction requires compensating free energy, which is provided in the assembled oligomer by numerous other hydrophobic contacts, such as van der Waals contacts. This balance of favorable and unfavorable forces is physiologically vital to produce a reversible protein-protein interaction. However, if the interfacial cavity is filled with an anesthetic, the balance of forces favors the oligomer to the point where reversibility might be compromised. This should increase the population (ie, concentration) of oligomers, which in some proteins, could trigger an oligomerization cascade (Fig. 5). In the case of amyloid β, these cavities are thought to be most prevalent in the diffusible oligomeric precursor of fibrils [73], the species also thought to be responsible for cytotoxicity.

Experimental evidence for the interaction

A simple way to measure oligomerization events is to monitor the increase in turbidity (ie, light scattering) in a sample as the aggregation events proceed. Using this approach, the authors found that the rate of amyloid β_{42} peptide oligomerization in vitro was dramatically increased in the presence of halothane (2-bromo-2-chloro-1,1,1-trifluoroethane) [74] (Fig. 6A). Significant acceleration of the aggregation was observed even at drug concentrations achieved in routine clinical anesthesia (<1.0 mM). Using electron microscopy, the sedimented material from these experiments was found to be fibrillar, similar to that found in Alzheimer senile plaque. In other experiments, the authors verified that a similar kinetic enhancement occurs with the more soluble amyloid β_{40} peptide, although on a longer time scale, as expected (data not shown). The cross-β fibrils characteristic of these neurodegenerative-disease-associated protein aggregates specifically bind the fluorescent dye, thioflavin-T (ThT), which then changes its

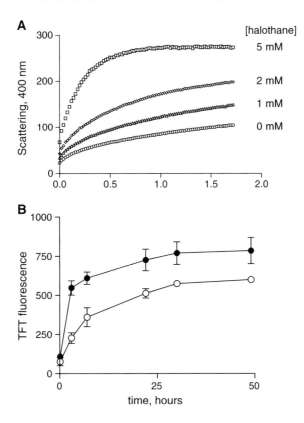

Fig. 6. (*A*) Incubation of amyloid β with various concentrations of halothane shows a dramatic increase in the rate of species that scatter visible light. Such species are typically quite large, so in this case probably indicate fibril formation. Even with clinical concentrations of halothane, a clear enhancement in rate of fibril formation is noted. (*B*) Using thioflavin T (TfT) binding to indicate cross-β oligomer formation, halothane is again noted to enhance the rate of a TfT binding species. (*From* Eckenhoff RG, Johansson JS, Wei H, et al. Inhaled anesthetic enhancement of amyloid-beta oligomerization and cytotoxicity. Anesthesiology 2004;101(3):705–6; with permission.)

emission characteristics dramatically. Thus, the authors also monitored aggregation of amyloid β using this approach, after first confirming that halothane had no effect on the fluorescence. The ThT fluorescence of amyloid $β_{42}$ samples was clearly enhanced in a time-dependent manner in the presence of halothane (Fig. 6B) consistent with the scattering data. These results were reproduced with the more commonly used anesthetic, isoflurane, although its oligomerization potency was somewhat less than halothane.It is crucial to know which of the many species of amyloid β oligomer the anesthetic favors. Clearly, the light scattering and ThT fluorescence assay mainly measure the formation of the mature fibril, the end product of the oligomerization cascade. The increase in rate of fibril formation could be achieved by the anesthetic preferring to bind to the fibril itself, or to intermediate oligomers. Since the latter is thought to be the toxic species, the difference is important. Thus, more recently, the authors have examined the differential binding using a variety of biophysical techniques. The distribution of oligomer sizes was measured using size-exclusion chromatography and analytical centrifugation. In both cases, volatile anesthetics were found to enhance the population of an intermediate oligomer of between 10 and 20 monomers. These experiments further suggested that the underlying biophysical mechanism was the lower solubility limit of the monomer, stemming from the volatile anesthetic, probably through a preferential interaction with the small oligomer (Fig. 7), which others have suggested have an abundance of cavities [73]. Further, the rank order of potency for lowering the threshold for oligomerization is consistent with our earlier work. That is, the potency of halothane is greater than that of isoflurane, which is greater than that of ethanol. Lowering of the oligomerization threshold has fundamental clinical implications. Because all people have some low concentration of amyloid β as a consequence of normal APP degradation, a lowering of the threshold for triggering the oligomerization cascade may initiate cytotoxicity and the pathogenesis of dementia earlier than would otherwise be the case. This is consistent with the clinical observations discussed below.

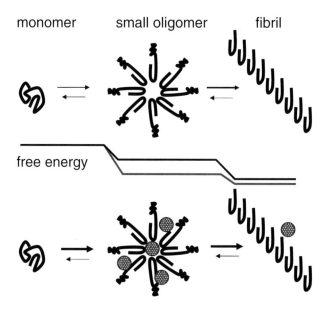

Fig. 7. The oligomerization cascade. Poorly structured monomer, on reaching a critical concentration, forms small homoligomers of between 5 and 20 monomers, the structure of which are not yet clear, but here indicated as an annular or micellar complex with a slightly helical character. These small, diffusible oligomers then form larger assemblies, gain more organized β structure, and ultimately form fibrils. There is some evidence that the small oligomers contain hydrophobic cavities, which might explain why anesthetics (shown here in dotted circles/line) appear to favor this species.

Halothane and isoflurane enhance pheochromocytoma-12 cytotoxicity in vitro

The above in vitro experiments confirm the general hypothesis, but do not necessarily indicate that anesthetics enhance the neurotoxicity of amyloid β. Experiments in a biological context are necessary to further confirm the notion. Thus, initially, the authors used a stable neuronal cell line, the pheochromocy-toma-12 line (PC-12), as a system to test the interaction between amyloid β and anesthetics. If general anesthetics increase the population of a toxic oligomer, then one would expect an increase in cell death when the cells were incubated with both protein and anesthetic. In the control experiments, PC-12 cells in-cubated with either halothane or isoflurane alone produced only small and insignificant changes in lactate dehydrogenase (LDH) release (Fig. 8). Fifteen μM amyloid β_{42} peptide alone produced a slightly greater increase in LDH, but the co-incubation of both anesthetic and amyloid β_{42} peptide resulted in a significant further increase in LDH release at both 1 and 2 minimum alveolar concentration. The rank order for cytotoxicity was similar to the above protein studies. That is, the cytotoxicity of isoflurane is greater than that of halothane, which is greater than that of propofol, which is greater than that of ethanol. In fact, the latter two compounds might confer a slight protective effect, although not statistically sig-nificant in the authors' experiments.

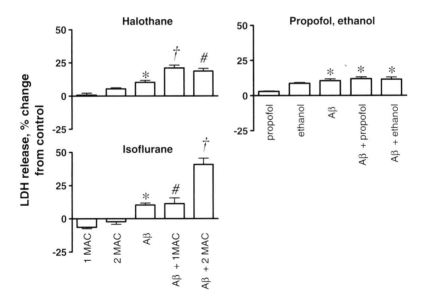

Fig. 8. The interaction between inhaled anesthetics and amyloid β_{42} (Aβ) is more toxic to PC-12 cells than the amyloid peptide alone, as indicated by the release of lactate dehydrogenase (LDH) 24 hours after a 6-hour exposure. On the other hand, neither propofol nor ethanol appears to enhance the cyto-toxicity of amyloid β. MAC, minimum alveolar concentration. (*From* Eckenhoff RG, Johansson JS, Wei H, et al. Inhaled anesthetic enhancement of amyloid-beta oligomerization and cytotoxicity. Anesthesiology 2004;101(3):707; with permission.)

Animal studies

Cells cannot adequately model intact organisms, so it is necessary to test these hypotheses on animals and, ultimately, people. However, to what extent can any animal species model neurodegenerative disorders? There does not appear to be naturally occurring impairment in any animal that is similar to Alzheimer's disease or Parkinson's disease. Thus, a variety of animal models have been developed to explore the molecular mechanisms underlying neurodegenerative disorders, including Alzheimer's disease, Parkinson's disease, Huntington's disease, frontal temporal dementia, and prion diseases. The authors review the currently available animal models of Alzheimer's disease, to reveal the strengths and limitations for testing the hypothesis for an interaction between anesthetics and neurodegeneration. Not a single published report on the effect of any anesthetic in any of the below animal models has appeared. The opportunities for further research are plentiful and the need for answers is enormous.

Invertebrate models

The nematode, *Caenorhabditis elegans,* and the fruit fly, *Drosophila melanogaster,* are unique models for the direct study of the mechanisms underlying Alzheimer's disease and other neurodegenerative diseases [75–77]. The experimental advantages include short life spans; well-characterized development, anatomy, and genetics; fully sequenced genomes; and clear anatomic endpoints (Fig. 9). Furthermore, fundamental features of the nervous systems are highly conserved between these invertebrates and humans, and the disruption of common cellular functions through protein misfolding and apoptosis may be similar. The modeling of Alzheimer's disease by the transgenic expression of human genes in invertebrates has provided important insights into the disease.

Amyloid β

Intracellular expression of the human amyloid β_{42} fragment in *C elegans* leads to adult onset paralysis, decreased life span [78], and intracellular accumulation of amyloid β aggregates (see Fig. 9) [79]. The worm Alzheimer's disease model revealed an up-regulation of chaperone proteins in cells expressing amyloid β [80], confirming the suspected role for misfolding in the pathogenesis. In *Drosophila,* the direct expression of both amyloid β_{42} and amyloid β_{40} causes progressive loss of learning ability, but amyloid β_{42} was found to have more significant age-dependent learning deficits, decreased life span, diffuse accumulations of amyloid-like plaques, and neuronal cell loss [81]. Targeted co-expression of human APP and β-secretase in another fly model [82] revealed immunoreactive amyloid β_{40} and amyloid β_{42} and age-dependent neurodegeneration in the retina in flies (see Fig. 9). These investigators also developed a triple-transgenic fly expressing APP, β-secretase, and presenilins. The fly was only able to survive if treated with β- or γ- secretase inhibitors. An increase in the activity of certain heat-shock proteins is neuroprotective in the fly. Thus, the

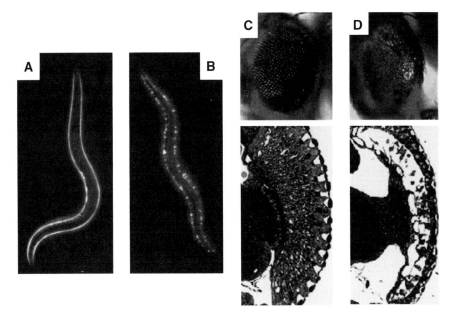

Fig. 9. Invertebrate models of neurodegenerative diseases. Panels *A* and *B* are fluorescence micrographs of the *C elegans* nematode transfected with either (*A*) normal green fluorescent protein (GFP), or (*B*) GFP linked with a 44-residue-long stretch of glutamine to simulate a Huntington's pathology. Note the aggregates of material easily visualized on fluorescence microscopy. Panels *C* and *D* are micrographs of a *Drosophila* eye, showing the retinal degeneration that results from targeted expression of amyloid or α-synuclein. The (*C*) upper and lower panels are of a normal eye, and the (*D*) upper and lower panels are from an animal with targeted expression of a polyglutamine containing protein. These endpoints in these simple creatures are easily monitored and quantitated using conventional techniques. (*Adapted from* Warrick JM, Chan HY, Chai Y, et al. Suppression of polyglutamine-mediated neurodegeneration in Drosophila by the molecular chaperone HSP70. Nat Genet 1999;23(4):426.)

disruption of protein folding or turnover may play a major role in neurodegenerative diseases [75,83].

Tau

C elegans [84] and *Drosophila* [84,85] models of tauopathy, produced by either expression of human tau or overexpression of a tau kinase, revealed the development of excessive tau phosphorylation, age-dependent neuronal degeneration, neuronal dysfunction, and accumulation of insoluble tau aggregates, but not the formation of neurofibrillary tangles. With the recent completion of the *C elegans* and *Drosophila* genomic sequence, the use of these invertebrate models to study isolated components of Alzheimer's disease has been invaluable in clarifying the underlying cellular mechanisms of this, and other, neurodegenerative diseases, as well as in providing candidate targets for therapeutics. The use of these simple models for anesthetic studies should lead rapidly to answers addressing specific hypotheses in intact organisms. For example, the above protein work suggests that anesthetics should enhance neuronal damage in both worm and fly models that produce amyloid β. Whether anesthetics interact with tau, or the associated kinases, is not yet clear, but these models represent ideal systems to initially address such questions and to refine hypotheses for testing in higher organisms.

Vertebrate models

Nontransgenic mouse models

The creation of a nontransgenic rodent model of amyloid pathology involves the exogenous (either intracerebroventricular or intraparenchymal) injection of amyloid β preparations in normal rodents [86]. The results indicate that the smaller diffusible form of amyloid β induces immediate but transient synaptic dysfunction because the injected material is rapidly cleared from the brain. Behavioral studies, however, show acute and transient deficits, including amnesia, after delivery of the soluble forms of amyloid β. Preparations of the larger fibrillar form of amyloid β also produces delayed memory impairment, possibly mediated by secondary processes, such as inflammatory and oxidative cascades, which have long-term effects on cellular function. The advantage of these nontransgenic models is that they allow one to directly examine the effects of the different isoforms of amyloid β over time, in different regions, and in different milieus, such as in the presence of anesthetics or other drugs. The disadvantage, of course, is the traumatic nature of delivery, and uncertain distribution and location.

APP transgenic mouse models

Several laboratories have produced animal models that overexpress the human form of APP. These transgenic mice exhibit Alzheimer's-disease-like pathology, including amyloid plaques, memory deficits, cell loss, and phosphorylated tau, but not neurofibrillary tangles. Although these models do not exhibit all of the hallmark features of Alzheimer's disease, they have provided valuable insight into the effects of amyloid β on brain pathology, behavior, and cognition [44,87].

The PDAPP transgenic mouse was the first model to produce pathology similar to Alzheimer's disease [88]. Mutant human APP (V717F) was expressed to produce human amyloid β_{42} and amyloid β_{40} at levels 5 to 14 times greater than the amyloid β produced by endogenous mouse APP. The phenotype included immunoreactive amyloid plaques in the cortex and hippocampus by around 1 year of age, gliosis and dystrophic neurons around the plaques, hyperphosphorylated tau proteins without neurofibrillary tangles, synaptic loss without concomitant neuronal loss, and brain region size reductions. Behaviorally, these mice exhibit memory impairment at 3 to 4 months of age, well before amyloid plaques could be detected [89]. The implication is that synaptotoxicity and neurotoxicity are related to the high levels of soluble or diffusible amyloid β, and not the insoluble fibrillar form, consistent with the discussion above.

The Tg2576 mouse model, which overexpresses the Swedish double mutant form of APP695 (K670N, M671L) [90], has been studied extensively. The mutations enhance APP degradation into amyloid β, and the promoters used cause mice brains to express about six times more mutant human APP than endogenous mouse APP. In addition to producing a similar Alzheimer's disease pathology as reported for the PDAPP mouse model, these transgenic mice developed cognitive deficits before the amyloid β plaques were detected, and in the absence of brain volumetric reductions or neuronal cell loss. This model is a step closer to resembling Alzheimer's disease, in that there is a steady decline in memory performance with increasing levels of insoluble amyloid β oligomers [91].

The APP23 mouse model expresses the same mutant human APP, but under a different promoter. The pathology and phenotype is similar to Tg2576 [92], but includes a severe cerebrovascular phenotype [93]. By 12 months of age, these mice have high levels of amyloid β and inflammation in the cerebral vasculature, resulting in progressive decrease in blood flow and microhemorrhages. This may therefore be a useful model of cerebrovasculitis (cerebral amyloid angiopathy) or hemorrhagic stroke [94], both of which are associated with a significant number of dementia cases. However, the cognitive changes observed in this animal model may result from impaired cerebral vascularization rather than the effects of APP or amyloid β on neuronal function.

The TgCRND8 mouse model [95] introduces another mutation in human APP to make a triple mutant form (K670N, M671L, V717I) using the same promoter as in Tg2576. This animal develops the phenotype earlier and in a more severe form. By 3 months, 50% die. Behavioral deficits are noted as early as 11 weeks in the Morris water maze [91]. The pathology includes plaques and dystrophic neurons initially in the cortex and hippocampus at 3 to 5 months of age and in other brain regions by 8 to 9 months.

Combined transgenic animals

In an attempt to produce mice with more pronounced and more rapidly developing Alzheimer's disease pathology, APP/PS1 double transgenic mouse models were developed [96–99]. These combine the Tg2576 human APP mutations with a M146L mutation in PS1. These transgenic mice exhibit cognitive impairment at 3 to 6 months and accelerated amyloid accumulation beginning at 3 months [100]. This is a departure from earlier work that demonstrated cognitive effects before plaque formation, which again suggests some neurotoxic role for the plaques themselves.

In yet another model expressing the Tg2576 gene, a knockout of the APP cleavage enzyme β-secretase [101] was included in an attempt to suppress the Tg2576 phenotype. Indeed, there was no detectable soluble amyloid β or plaques in this animal, and only mild behavioral deficits. This research establishes β-secretase as a potential therapeutic drug target and, together with the many other APP processing enzymes, a potential target for anesthetic actions.

From the animal models discussed above, considerable information on the role of amyloid β and APP in the development of neurodegenerative pathologies has accrued. However, unlike Alzheimer's disease in the human, none of these models develop tau pathology or significant neurodegeneration and brain volume reduction. An initial attempt to combine amyloid and tau pathology by crossing mutant APP and mutant tau mice resulted in a mouse with more neurofibrillary tangles than singly transgenic tau mice [102], but, interestingly, without amyloid β plaques. That amyloid β and tau interact is also demonstrated by enhanced tau pathology after direct injection of amyloid β into tau mutant mice [53]. This represents yet another protein-protein interaction that anesthetics might modulate.

Triple transgenic mouse model

Recently, a triple-transgenic mouse model (3xTg-AD) has been produced that combines mutations in APP, tau, and PS1 [44]. This mouse progressively develops both amyloid β and tau pathologies and the phenotype closely mimics that of human Alzheimer's disease. Extracellular amyloid β deposits form around 6 months of age and tau neurofibrillary tangles form at 10 to 12 months of age (Fig. 10)

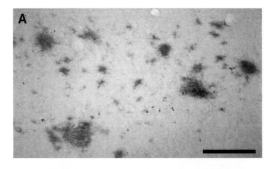

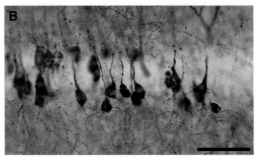

Fig. 10. Light micrographs from the recent triple-transgenic mouse model of Alzheimer's disease. Note similarity of these plaques (*A*) and neurofibrillary tangles (*B*) to those related to the human disorder, shown in Fig. 2. (*From* LaFerla FM, Oddo S. Alzheimer's disease: Abeta, tau and synaptic dysfunction. Trends Mol Med 2005;11(4):173.)

[103]. Furthermore, the tau protein undergoes an early conformational change followed by hyperphosphorylation at the same specific residues as in human Alzheimer's disease. Behavioral studies in the 3xTg-AD mice demonstrated age-dependent cognitive deficits that temporally correlated with an accumulation of intraneuronal amyloid β, which precedes amyloid β plaque and neurofibrillary tangle pathology [104]. Intraneuronal amyloid β has also been associated with synaptic dysfunction [103], suggesting that cognitive decline and synaptic dysfunction are early events in Alzheimer's disease pathology. New evidence suggests that intermediate amyloid β oligomers accumulate intraneuronally, and that amyloid β oligomers may play a role in the induction of tau pathology [67]. This observation in an intact animal model returns us full circle to the notion that amyloid β oligomerization is the pivotal step in the progression of neuro-degenerative disorders, and highlights our observation that anesthetics appear to favor this step.

Human studies

The authors have alluded above to the potential interaction between neuro-degeneration and anesthesia, and yet animal data are yet to appear. Is there clinical evidence of an association? Certainly, anesthesia and surgery have long been suspected of producing cognitive problems [5,7,8], a suspicion recently confirmed in several human studies. This effect, now called postoperative cognitive dysfunction, is most common in the elderly, although it is also documented in the middle aged, and it is suspected to exist in the very young. Although it has never been clear that anesthesia per se is responsible, recent animal studies suggest that certain inhaled anesthetics can independently produce long-term learning and memory defects [105–107]. In addition to these documented effects on learning and memory, the interaction between prior surgery and neurodegenerative disorders, such as Alzheimer's disease, has been examined in a few small studies [108,109]. One study found an association between the number of prior anesthetics and the age of Alzheimer's disease diagnosis in a group of 252 patients (no controls) with established Alzheimer's disease [110]. Researchers found that larger numbers of anesthetics before age 50 predicted an earlier onset of Alzheimer's disease. Recognizing the limitations of this initial work, the same researchers conducted another study where the Alzheimer's disease patients where matched with controls [108]. Although the odds ratios for an association between prior anesthesia and Alzheimer's disease did not reach statistical significance, the point estimates all indicated an effect, and there appears to be a dose-response relationship (Fig. 11). Another study with 115 Alzheimer's disease patients and matched controls (All controls had some form of neurological disorder.), found a 1.78:1 odds ratio for an association between the number of anesthetics in the 5 years before Alzheimer's disease diagnosis as compared with the control group [111]. Again, this odds ratio did not reach statistical significance. However, the estimates from all three studies are positive, and of roughly

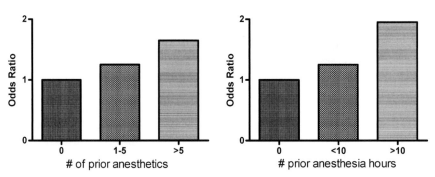

Fig. 11. Relative risk (odds ratio) of acquiring Alzheimer's disease as a function of the number of prior anesthetics (*left*) and as a function of the cumulative number of hours of anesthesia (*right*). Although the differences in these data do not reach statistical significance, the dose-response trend is of interest and hardly comforting. (*Data from* Bohnen N, Warner MA, Kokmen E, et al. Alzheimer's disease and cumulative exposure to anesthesia: a case-control study. J Am Geriatr Soc 1994;42(2):200.)

the same magnitude. Finally, a recent retrospective cohort study reported an almost twofold increase in risk of developing Alzheimer's disease following coronary artery bypass surgery as compared with percutaneous transluminal coronary angioplasty [112]. This effect did reach statistical significance, but it is difficult to attribute the effect to any specific feature of the two procedures. Nevertheless, there are differences in the anesthetic exposure between the two procedures. Coronary artery bypass surgery patients receive both narcotics and inhaled anesthetics, while the percutaneous transluminal coronary angioplasty patients typically receive intravenous sedative hypnotics (eg, benzodiazepines, propofol). Thus, while the accumulated evidence for an association between surgery requiring anesthesia and Alzheimer's disease remains weak, the consistent positive odds ratio of between 1.4:1 and 1.9:1 in the face of underpowered retrospective studies, do not give confidence for an absence of risk. A therapeutic with a similar magnitude of effect in the opposite direction would be hailed as a breakthrough. Thus, the data from these studies cannot be discounted yet because of statistical or design issues. Further investigation at both the clinical and basic science level seems warranted to rapidly assess both the magnitude and mechanism of an effect.

Summary

The prevalence of the neurodegenerative disorders is increasing as life expectancy lengthens, and there exists concern that environmental influences may contribute to this increase. These disorders are varied in their clinical presentation, but appear to have a common biophysical initiation. At this level, it is both plausible and now proven that anesthetics can enhance aggregation of some disease-causing proteins. Although data in support of an interaction in animal models are still lacking, data from clinical studies indicate an association, which provides further cause for concern. Many opportunities exist for rapid progress at all levels on defining whether anesthetics do indeed contribute to the pathogenesis of these progressive, debilitating disorders.

References

[1] Hebert LE, Scherr PA, Bienias JL, et al. Alzheimer disease in the US population: prevalence estimates using the 2000 census. Arch Neurol 2003;60(8):1119–22.

[2] Small GW, Rabins PV, Barry PP, et al. Diagnosis and treatment of Alzheimer disease and related disorders. Consensus statement of the American Association for Geriatric Psychiatry, the Alzheimer's Association, and the American Geriatrics Society. JAMA 1997;278(16):1363–71.

[3] Tanner CM, Goldman SM. Epidemiology of Parkinson's disease. Neurol Clin 1996;14(2):317–35.

[4] Albers JW, Wald JJ, Trask CL, et al. Evaluation of blink reflex results obtained from workers previously diagnosed with solvent-induced toxic encephalopathy. J Occup Environ Med 2001; 43(8):713–22.

[5] Moller JT, Cluitmans P, Rasmussen LS, et al. Long-term postoperative cognitive dysfunction in the elderly ISPOCD1 study. ISPOCD investigators. International Study of Post-Operative Cognitive Dysfunction. [Erratum appears in Lancet 1998;351(9117):1742]. Lancet 1998;351(9106): 857–61.

[6] Nishikawa K, Nakayama M, Omote K, et al. Recovery characteristics and post-operative delirium after long-duration laparoscope-assisted surgery in elderly patients: propofol-based vs. sevoflurane-based anesthesia. Acta Anaesthesiol Scand 2004;48:162–8.

[7] Ancelin ML, de Roquefeuil G, Ledesert B, et al. Exposure to anaesthetic agents, cognitive functioning and depressive symptomatology in the elderly. Br J Psychiatry 2001;178:360–6.

[8] Johnson T, Monk T, Rasmussen LS, et al. Postoperative cognitive dysfunction in middle-aged patients. Anesthesiology 2002;96(6):1351–7.

[9] Bedford PD. Adverse cerebral effects of anesthesia on old people. Lancet 1955;ii:259–63.

[10] Breteler MM, Claus JJ, van Duijn CM, et al. Epidemiology of Alzheimer's disease. Epidemiol Rev 1992;14:59–82.

[11] Kawas CH, Katzman R. Epidemiology of Dementia and Alzheimer Disease. In: Terry RD, Katzman R, Bick KL, et al, editors. Alzheimer Disease. Philadelphia: Lippincott Williams & Wilkins; 1999. p. 95–116.

[12] Stromer T, Serpell LC. Structure and morphology of the Alzheimer's amyloid fibril. Microsc Res Tech 2005;67(3–4):210–7.

[13] Seabrook GR, Smith DW, Bowery BJ, et al. Mechanisms contributing to the deficits in hippocampal synaptic plasticity in mice lacking amyloid precursor protein. Neuropharmacol 1999; 38(3):349–59.

[14] Muller U, Cristina N, Li ZW, et al. Behavioral and anatomical deficits in mice homozygous for a modified beta-amyloid precursor protein gene. Cell 1994;79(5):755–65.

[15] Zheng H, Jiang M, Trumbauer ME, et al. beta-Amyloid precursor protein-deficient mice show reactive gliosis and decreased locomotor activity. Cell 1995;81(4):525–31.

[16] Hardy J, Selkoe DJ. The amyloid hypothesis of Alzheimer's disease: progress and problems on the road to therapeutics. [Erratum appears in Science 2002;297(5590):2209]. Science 2002; 297(5580):353–6.

[17] Terry RD, Masliah E, Hansen LL. The neuropathology of Alzheimer disease and the structural basis of its cognitive alterations. In: Terry RD, Katzman R, Bick KL, et al, editors. Alzheimer Disease. Philadelphia: Lippincott Williams and Wilkins; 1999. p. 187–206.

[18] Klein WL, Krafft GA, Finch CE. Targeting small Abeta oligomers: the solution to an Alzheimer's disease conundrum? Trends Neurosci 2001;24(4):219–24.

[19] Kayed R, Head E, Thompson JL, et al. Common structure of soluble amyloid oligomers implies common mechanism of pathogenesis. Science 2003;300(5618):486–9.

[20] Klein WL, Stine Jr WB, Teplow DB. Small assemblies of unmodified amyloid beta-protein are the proximate neurotoxin in Alzheimer's disease. Neurobiol Aging 2004;25(5):569–80.

[21] Glabe CG, Kayed R. Common structure and toxic function of amyloid oligomers implies a common mechanism of pathogenesis. Neurology 2005. Available at: http://www.ncbi.nlm.nih. gov/entrez/query.fcgi?cmd=Retrieve&db=pubmed&dopt=Abstract&list_uids=16361390&itool= iconabstr&query_hl=13&itool=pubmed_docsum. Accessed February 27, 2006.

[22] Muchowski PJ, Wacker JL. Modulation of neurodegeneration by molecular chaperones. Nat Rev Neurosci 2005;6(1):11–22.

[23] Auluck PK, Meulener MC, Bonini NM. Mechanisms of suppression of α-synuclein neurotoxicity by geldanamycin in Drosophila. J Biol Chem 2005;280(4):2873–8.

[24] Wisniewski T, Frangione B. Immunological and anti-chaperone therapeutic approaches for Alzheimer disease. Brain Pathol 2005;15(1):72–7.

[25] Bayer AJ, Bullock R, Jones RW, et al. Evaluation of the safety and immunogenicity of synthetic Abeta42 (AN1792) in patients with AD. Neurology 2005;64(1):94–101.

[26] Schenk D, Hagen M, Seubert P. Current progress in beta-amyloid immunotherapy. Curr Opin Immunol 2004;16(5):599–606.

[27] Schenk D, Barbour R, Dunn W, et al. Immunization with amyloid-beta attenuates Alzheimerdisease-like pathology in the PDAPP mouse. Nature 1999;400(6740):173–7.

[28] Weiner HL, Lemere CA, Maron R, et al. Nasal administration of amyloid-beta peptide decreases cerebral amyloid burden in a mouse model of Alzheimer's disease. Ann Neurol 2000; 48(4):567–79.

[29] Janus C, Pearson J, McLaurin J, et al. A beta peptide immunization reduces behavioural impairment and plaques in a model of Alzheimer's disease. Nature 2000;408(6815):979–82.

[30] Jensen MT, Mottin MD, Cracchiolo JR, et al. Lifelong immunization with human beta-amyloid (1–42) protects Alzheimer's transgenic mice against cognitive impairment throughout aging. Neuroscience 2005;130(3):667–84.

[31] Lemere CA, Beierschmitt A, Iglesias M, et al. Alzheimer's disease abeta vaccine reduces central nervous system abeta levels in a non-human primate, the Caribbean vervet. Am J Pathol 2004;165(1):283–97.

[32] Bard F, Cannon C, Barbour R, et al. Peripherally administered antibodies against amyloid betapeptide enter the central nervous system and reduce pathology in a mouse model of Alzheimer disease. Nat Med 2000;6(8):916–9.

[33] DeMattos RB, Bales KR, Cummins DJ, et al. Peripheral anti-A beta antibody alters CNS and plasma A beta clearance and decreases brain A beta burden in a mouse model of Alzheimer's disease. Proc Natl Acad Sci USA 2001;98(15):8850–5.

[34] Oddo S, Billings L, Kesslak JP, et al. Abeta immunotherapy leads to clearance of early, but not late, hyperphosphorylated tau aggregates via the proteasome. Neuron 2004;43(3): 321–32.

[35] McLaurin J, Cecal R, Kierstead ME, et al. Therapeutically effective antibodies against amyloidbeta peptide target amyloid-beta residues 4–10 and inhibit cytotoxicity and fibrillogenesis. Nat Med 2002;8(11):1263–9.

[36] Oddo S, Caccamo A, Smith I, et al. A dynamic relationship between intracellular and extracellular pools of aβ. Am J Pathol 2006;168(1):184–94.

[37] Morgan D, Diamond DM, Gottschall PE, et al. A beta peptide vaccination prevents memory loss in an animal model of Alzheimer's disease. [Erratum appears in Nature 2001;412(6847):660]. Nature 2000;408(6815):982–5.

[38] Kotilinek LA, Bacskai B, Westerman M, et al. Reversible memory loss in a mouse transgenic model of Alzheimer's disease. J Neurosci 2002;22(15):6331–5.

[39] Senior K. Dosing in phase II trial of Alzheimer's vaccine suspended. Lancet Neurol 2002; 1(1):3.

[40] Orgogozo JM, Gilman S, Dartigues JF, et al. Subacute meningoencephalitis in a subset of patients with AD after Abeta42 immunization. Neurology 2003;61(1):46–54.

[41] Michaelis ML. Drugs targeting Alzheimer's disease: some things old and some things new. J Pharmacol Exp Ther 2003;304(3):897–904.

[42] De Felice FG, Vieira MN, Saraiva LM, et al. Targeting the neurotoxic species in Alzheimer's disease: inhibitors of Abeta oligomerization. FASEB J 2004;18(12):1366−72.

[43] Lashuel HA, Hartley DM, Balakhaneh D, et al. New class of inhibitors of amyloid-beta fibril formation. Implications for the mechanism of pathogenesis in Alzheimer's disease. J Biol Chem 2002;277(45):42881−90.

[44] LaFerla FM, Oddo S. Alzheimer's disease: Abeta, tau and synaptic dysfunction. Trends Mol Med 2005;11(4):170−6.

[45] Binder LI, Guillozet-Bongaarts AL, Garcia-Sierra F, et al. Tau, tangles, and Alzheimer's disease. Biochim Biophys Acta 2005;1739(2−3):216−23.

[46] Lee VM, Goedert M, Trojanowski JQ. Neurodegenerative tauopathies. Annu Rev Neurosci 2001;24:1121−59.

[47] Forman MS, Trojanowski JQ, Lee VM. Neurodegenerative diseases: a decade of discoveries paves the way for therapeutic breakthroughs. Nat Med 2004;10(10):1055−63.

[48] Kotzbauer PT, Trojanowsk JQ, Lee VM. Lewy body pathology in Alzheimer's disease. J Mol Neurosci 2001;17(2):225−32.

[49] Goedert M. Alpha-synuclein and neurodegenerative diseases. Nat Rev Neurosci 2001;2(7): 492−501.

[50] Norris EH, Giasson BI, Lee VM. Alpha-synuclein: normal function and role in neurodegenerative diseases. Curr Top Dev Biol 2004;60:17−54.

[51] Bennett MC. The role of alpha-synuclein in neurodegenerative diseases. Pharmacol Ther 2005; 105(3):311−31.

[52] Masliah E, Rockenstein E, Veinbergs I, et al. Beta-amyloid peptides enhance alpha-synuclein accumulation and neuronal deficits in a transgenic mouse model linking Alzheimer's disease and Parkinson's disease. Proc Natl Acad Sci USA 2001;98(21):12245−50.

[53] Gotz J, Chen F, van Dorpe J, et al. Formation of neurofibrillary tangles in P301l tau transgenic mice induced by Abeta 42 fibrils. Science 2001;293(5534):1491−5.

[54] Giasson BI, Forman MS, Higuchi M, et al. Initiation and synergistic fibrillization of tau and alpha-synuclein. Science 2003;300(5619):636−40.

[55] Kotzbauer PT, Giasson BI, Kravitz AV, et al. Fibrillization of alpha-synuclein and tau in familial Parkinson's disease caused by the A53T alpha-synuclein mutation. Exp Neurol 2004;187(2): 279−88.

[56] Frasier M, Wolozin B. Following the leader: fibrillization of alpha-synuclein and tau. Exp Neurol 2004;187(2):235−9.

[57] Zoghbi HY, Orr HT. Glutamine repeats and neurodegeneration. Annu Rev Neurosci 2000;23: 217−47.

[58] Weissmann C. The state of the prion. Nat Rev Microbiol 2004;2(11):861−71.

[59] DeArmond SJ, Prusiner SB. Perspectives on prion biology, prion disease pathogenesis, and pharmacologic approaches to treatment. Clin Lab Med 2003;23(1):1−41.

[60] Prusiner SB, Scott MR, DeArmond SJ, et al. Prion protein biology. Cell 1998;93(3):337−48.

[61] Stefani M, Dobson CM. Protein aggregation and aggregate toxicity: new insights into protein folding, misfolding diseases and biological evolution. J Mol Med 2003;81(11):678−99.

[62] Dobson CM. Protein folding and misfolding. Nature 2003;426(6968):884−90.

[63] Selkoe DJ. Cell biology of protein misfolding: the examples of Alzheimer's and Parkinson's diseases. Nat Cell Biol 2004;6(11):1054−61.

[64] Bucciantini M, Calloni G, Chiti F, et al. Prefibrillar amyloid protein aggregates share common features of cytotoxicity. J Biol Chem 2004;279(30):31374−82.

[65] Petkova AT, Ishii Y, Balbach JJ, et al. A structural model for Alzheimer's beta-amyloid fibrils based on experimental constraints from solid state NMR. Proc Natl Acad Sci USA 2002;99(26): 16742−7.

[66] Kanno T, Yamaguchi K, Naiki H, et al. Association of thin filaments into thick filaments revealing the structural hierarchy of amyloid fibrils. J Struct Biol 2005;149(2):213−8.

[67] Oddo S, Caccamo A, Tran L, et al. Temporal profile of Abeta oligomerization in an in vivo model of Alzheimer's disease: a link between Abeta and tau pathology. J Biol Chem 2006; 281(3):1599−604.

[68] Eckenhoff RG, Johansson JS. Molecular interactions between inhaled anesthetics and proteins. Pharmacol Rev 1997;49(4):343–67.

[69] Eckenhoff RG, Petersen CE, Ha CE, et al. Inhaled anesthetic binding sites in human serum albumin. J Biol Chem 2000;275(39):30439–44.

[70] Kutchai H, Geddis LM, Jones LR, et al. Differential effects of general anesthetics on the quaternary structure of the Ca-ATPases of cardiac and skeletal sarcoplasmic reticulum. Biochemistry 1998;37(8):2410–21.

[71] Eckenhoff RG, Pidikiti R, Reddy KS. Anesthetic stabilization of protein intermediates: myoglobin and halothane. Biochemistry 2001;40(36):10819–24.

[72] Hubbard SJ, Argos P. Cavities and packing at protein interfaces. Protein Sci 1994;3(12): 2194–206.

[73] Chatani E, Goto Y. Structural stability of amyloid fibrils of beta(2)-microglobulin in comparison with its native fold. Biochim Biophys Acta 2005;1753(1):64–75.

[74] Eckenhoff RG, Johansson JS, Wei H, et al. Inhaled anesthetic enhancement of amyloid-beta oligomerization and cytotoxicity. Anesthesiology 2004;101(3):703–9.

[75] Link CD. Invertebrate models of Alzheimer's disease. Genes Brain Behav 2005;4(3):147–56.

[76] Bilen J, Bonini NM. Drosophila as a model for human neurodegenerative disease. Annu Rev Genet 2005;39:153–71.

[77] Warrick JM, Chan HY, Chai Y, et al. Suppression of polyglutamine-mediated neurodegeneration in Drosophila by the molecular chaperone HSP70. Nat Genet 1999;23(4):425–8.

[78] Link CD. Expression of human beta-amyloid peptide in transgenic Caenorhabditis elegans. Proc Natl Acad Sci USA 1995;92(20):9368–72.

[79] Link CD, Johnson CJ, Fonte V, et al. Visualization of fibrillar amyloid deposits in living, transgenic Caenorhabditis elegans animals using the sensitive amyloid dye, X-34. Neurobiol Aging 2001;22(2):217–26.

[80] Link CD, Taft A, Kapulkin V, et al. Gene expression analysis in a transgenic Caenorhabditis elegans Alzheimer's disease model. Neurobiol Aging 2003;24(3):397–413.

[81] Iijima K, Liu HP, Chiang AS, et al. Dissecting the pathological effects of human Abeta40 and Abeta42 in Drosophila: a potential model for Alzheimer's disease. Proc Natl Acad Sci USA 2004;101(17):6623–8.

[82] Greeve I, Kretzschmar D, Tschape JA, et al. Age-dependent neurodegeneration and Alzheimer-amyloid plaque formation in transgenic Drosophila. J Neurosci 2004;24(16):3899–906.

[83] Auluck PK, Chan HY, Trojanowski JQ, et al. Chaperone suppression of alpha-synuclein toxicity in a Drosophila model for Parkinson's disease. Science 2002;295(5556):865–8.

[84] Nishimura I, Yang Y, Lu B. PAR-1 kinase plays an initiator role in a temporally ordered phosphorylation process that confers tau toxicity in Drosophila. Cell 2004;116(5):671–82.

[85] Jackson GR, Wiedau-Pazos M, Sang TK, et al. Human wild-type tau interacts with wingless pathway components and produces neurofibrillary pathology in Drosophila. Neuron 2002; 34(4):509–19.

[86] Stephan A, Phillips AG. A case for a non-transgenic animal model of Alzheimer's disease. Genes Brain Behav 2005;4(3):157–72.

[87] Kobayashi DT, Chen KS. Behavioral phenotypes of amyloid-based genetically modified mouse models of Alzheimer's disease. Genes Brain Behav 2005;4(3):173–96.

[88] Games D, Adams D, Alessandrini R, et al. Alzheimer-type neuropathology in transgenic mice overexpressing V717F beta-amyloid precursor protein. Nature 1995;373(6514):523–7.

[89] Chen G, Chen KS, Knox J, et al. A learning deficit related to age and beta-amyloid plaques in a mouse model of Alzheimer's disease. Nature 2000;408(6815):975–9.

[90] Hsiao K, Chapman P, Nilsen S, et al. Correlative memory deficits, Abeta elevation, and amyloid plaques in transgenic mice. Science 1996;274(5284):99–102.

[91] Westerman MA, Cooper-Blacketer D, Mariash A, et al. The relationship between Abeta and memory in the Tg2576 mouse model of Alzheimer's disease. J Neurosci 2002;22(5): 1858–67.

[92] Van Dam D, D'Hooge R, Staufenbiel M, et al. Age-dependent cognitive decline in the APP23 model precedes amyloid deposition. Eur J Neurosci 2003;17(2):388–96.

[93] Sturchler-Pierrat C, Abramowski D, Duke M, et al. Two amyloid precursor protein transgenic mouse models with Alzheimer disease-like pathology. Proc Natl Acad Sci USA 1997;94(24): 13287–92.

[94] Winkler DT, Bondolfi L, Herzig MC, et al. Spontaneous hemorrhagic stroke in a mouse model of cerebral amyloid angiopathy. J Neurosci 2001;21(5):1619–27.

[95] Chishti MA, Yang DS, Janus C, et al. Early-onset amyloid deposition and cognitive deficits in transgenic mice expressing a double mutant form of amyloid precursor protein 695. J Biol Chem 2001;276(24):21562–70.

[96] Holcomb L, Gordon MN, McGowan E, et al. Accelerated Alzheimer-type phenotype in transgenic mice carrying both mutant amyloid precursor protein and presenilin 1 transgenes. Nat Med 1998;4(1):97–100.

[97] Arendash GW, King DL, Gordon MN, et al. Progressive, age-related behavioral impairments in transgenic mice carrying both mutant amyloid precursor protein and presenilin-1 transgenes. Brain Res 2001;891(1–2):42–53.

[98] McGowan E, Sanders S, Iwatsubo T, et al. Amyloid phenotype characterization of transgenic mice overexpressing both mutant amyloid precursor protein and mutant presenilin 1 transgenes. Neurobiol Dis 1999;6(4):231–44.

[99] Kurt MA, Davies DC, Kidd M, et al. Neurodegenerative changes associated with beta-amyloid deposition in the brains of mice carrying mutant amyloid precursor protein and mutant presenilin-1 transgenes. Exp Neurol 2001;171(1):59–71.

[100] Howlett DR, Richardson JC, Austin A, et al. Cognitive correlates of Abeta deposition in male and female mice bearing amyloid precursor protein and presenilin-1 mutant transgenes. Brain Res 2004;1017(1–2):130–6.

[101] Ohno M, Sametsky EA, Younkin LH, et al. BACE1 deficiency rescues memory deficits and cholinergic dysfunction in a mouse model of Alzheimer's disease. Neuron 2004;41(1):27–33.

[102] Lewis J, McGowan E, Rockwood J, et al. Neurofibrillary tangles, amyotrophy and progressive motor disturbance in mice expressing mutant (P301L) tau protein. [Erratum appears in Nat Genet 2000;26(1):127]. Nat Genet 2000;25(4):401–5.

[103] Oddo S, Caccamo A, Shepherd JD, et al. Triple-transgenic model of Alzheimer's disease with plaques and tangles: intracellular Abeta and synaptic dysfunction. Neuron 2003;39(3):409–21.

[104] Billings LM, Oddo S, Green KN, et al. Intraneuronal Abeta causes the onset of early Alzheimer's disease-related cognitive deficits in transgenic mice. Neuron 2005;45(5):675–88.

[105] Culley DJ, Baxter MG, Crosby CA, et al. Impaired acquisition of spatial memory 2 weeks after isoflurane and isoflurane-nitrous oxide anesthesia in aged rats. Anesth Analg 2004;99(5): 1393–7.

[106] Jevtovic-Todorovic V, Hartman RE, Izumi Y, et al. Early exposure to common anesthetic agents causes widespread neurodegeneration in the developing rat brain and persistent learning deficits. J Neurosci 2003;23(3):876–82.

[107] Jevtovic-Todorovic V, Carter LB. The anesthetics nitrous oxide and ketamine are more neurotoxic to old than to young rat brain. Neurobiol Aging 2005;26(6):947–56.

[108] Bohnen N, Warner MA, Kokmen E, et al. Alzheimer's disease and cumulative exposure to anesthesia: a case-control study. J Am Geriatr Soc 1994;42(2):198–201.

[109] Muravchick S, Smith DS. Parkinsonian symptoms during emergence from general anesthesia. Anesthesiology 1995;82(1):305–7.

[110] Bohnen N, Warner MA, Kokmen E, et al. Early and midlife exposure to anesthesia and age of onset of Alzheimer's disease. Intern J Neurosci 1994;77(3–4):181–5.

[111] Gasparini M, Vanacore N, Schiaffini C, et al. A case-control study on Alzheimer's disease and exposure to anesthesia. Neurol Sci 2002;23(1):11–4.

[112] Lee TA, Wolozin B, Weiss KB, et al. Assessment of the emergence of Alzheimer's disease following coronary artery bypass graft surgery or percutaneous transluminal coronary angioplasty. J Alzheimers Dis 2005;7(4):319–24.

ELSEVIER
SAUNDERS

Anesthesiology Clin N Am
24 (2006) 407–417

ANESTHESIOLOGY
CLINICS OF
NORTH AMERICA

The Impact of Intraoperative Monitoring on Patient Safety

James B. Mayfield, MD

*Department of Anesthesiology and Perioperative Medicine, Medical College of Georgia,
1150 15th Street, BIW 2144, Augusta, GA 30912-2700, USA*

A common goal among physicians and nurses who practice anesthesia is to make surgery and anesthesia as safe as possible. In the modern practice of anesthesiology, many different monitors are used to acquire essential information to enhance patient care. We routinely rely on sophisticated monitors to ensure adequate function of anesthesia machines and assess physiologic function and depth of anesthesia. The question as to whether any of our intraoperative monitors have impact on patient safety has gained considerable attention in recent years. Physicians monitor patients to recognize and evaluate potential physiologic problems and identify prognostic trends. Although it is rational to believe that improved monitoring should reduce risk and increase patient safety, we must look critically at the evidence.

A common goal among physicians and nurses who practice anesthesia is to make surgery and anesthesia as safe as possible. In the modern practice of anesthesiology, many different monitors are used to acquire essential information to enhance patient care. We routinely rely on sophisticated monitors to ensure adequate function of anesthesia machines and assess physiologic function and depth of anesthesia. The question as to whether any of our intraoperative monitors have impact on patient safety has gained considerable attention in recent years. Physicians monitor patients to recognize and evaluate potential physiologic problems and identify prognostic trends. Although it is rational to believe that improved monitoring should reduce risk and increase patient safety, we must look critically at the evidence.

E-mail address: jmayfield@mcg.edu

Anesthesia monitoring standards from a historical perspective

Understanding the historical events behind anesthesia safety initiatives allows us to look critically at the impact that anesthesia monitors have had on patient safety. In 1954, a huge controversy surrounded the publication by Beecher and Todd [1] of an article entitled "A Study of the Deaths Associated with Anesthesia and Surgery." Beecher examined almost 600,000 anesthetics administered over a 5-year period at ten university hospitals. He found the incidence of mortality in which anesthesia was the primary cause to be 3.7 per 10,000. In the following years, several other studies came to similar conclusions. Dripps [2] analyzed approximately 33,000 records at the University of Pennsylvania and found an overall mortality with anesthesia as the primary cause at 11.7 per 10,000 anesthetics. Phillips and colleagues [3] studied anesthetics given over a 5.5-year period in Baltimore and found anesthesia to be the principal cause of mortality in approximately 6% of cases. More recently, major reports concerning anesthesia-related mortality have come from international sources. In 1982, Lunn and Mushin [4] reported on data from the United Kingdom. They found the anesthesia-related mortality rate to be 1 to 2 per 10,000. They also noted that large numbers of patients did not have intraoperative blood pressure or electrocardiographic monitoring. Although the results of these morbidity studies were debated over many years within the anesthesia community, the most important result of these studies was the dramatic drive among anesthesiologists to improve anesthesia quality and outcome.

Before the 1980s, little national attention was given to the concept of standard patient monitoring to increase safety and decrease morbidity. Most anesthesiologists would practice as they had been taught. In 1985, however, several groups began to develop monitoring standards with the hope of early detection of untoward patient trends or events during anesthesia. It was thought that in preventing patient injury, the explosive increases in anesthesia-related malpractice actions, judgments, and insurance premiums could be halted. One of the first such groups was the Arizona Society of Anesthesiologists, who developed "Guidelines for Patient Care in Anesthesiology" [5]. These guidelines included the use of the following:

1. Oxygen analyzer with low concentration alarm
2. Anesthesia ventilator low-pressure alarm
3. Two of the following modalities: noninvasive or continuous blood pressure monitor, continuous electrocardiographic display, or precordial esophageal stethoscope

On March 25, 1985, the Department of Anesthesia of the Harvard Medical School adopted its "Standards of Practice 1: Minimal Monitoring" [6]. This standard was for all patients who received general, regional, or monitored anesthesia care at all designated anesthetizing locations, unless it was clinically impractical. The standards are listed in Box 1.

Box 1. Harvard Medical School standards of patient monitoring

- Blood pressure and heart rate recorded at least every 5 minutes
- Continuous electrocardiogram throughout case
- Continuous monitoring of ventilation and circulation by at least one of the following:
  Ventilation
      a. Observation of the reservoir breathing bag
      b. Auscultation of breath sounds
  Circulation
      a. Intra-arterial pressure monitoring
      b. Pulse plethysmography
      c. Ultrasound peripheral pulse monitoring
- Breathing system disconnect monitor with alarm
- Oxygen analyzer with low concentration alarm
- Temperature measurement

Adapted from Eichhorn JH, Cooper JR, Cullen DJ, et al. Standards for patient monitoring during anesthesia at Harvard Medical School. JAMA 1986;256:1017–20.

With the publication of these new standards, the anesthesia community entered a new era. An expectation of future national standards with an increasing uniformity of anesthesia practice was on the horizon. In 1985, the Anesthesia Patient Safety Foundation was created to raise the levels of consciousness and knowledge of patient safety issues. In early 1986, the American Society of Anesthesiology was the first medical specialty to adopt standards of care for its members [7].

Professional liability effects on patient monitoring

The first international symposium on preventable anesthesia mortality and morbidity was held in Boston in 1984 [8]. At that conference, preliminary findings that examined closed malpractice claims against anesthesiologists in the state of Washington were presented. Because anesthesiologists nationwide were facing huge malpractice insurance premiums, leadership of the American Society of Anesthesiology began a national closed claims analysis under the direction of Fred Cheney, chairman of the American Society of Anesthesiology committee on professional liability. Cheney noted, "The relationship of patient safety to malpractice insurance premiums was easy to predict. If patients were not injured, they would not sue, and if the payout for anesthesia related patient injury could be reduced then insurance rates would follow" [9]. It was hoped that the com-

bination of standards of care, with regards to patient monitoring and an examination of the closed claims against anesthesiologists, would lead to a better
understanding in the prevention of poor outcomes and significantly lower malpractice premiums.

In mid-1980s to early 1990s, the pulse oximeter and end tidal carbon dioxide
capnograph monitors came into widespread use. Analysis of the data obtained in
the 1990s compared with the 1980s shows significant differences in respiratory
events. The most common respiratory events that caused permanent brain damage
or death were inadequate ventilation, esophageal intubation, and difficult intubation. Claims for inadequate ventilation and esophageal intubation were 25% of
the claims for brain damage or death in the 1980s. This number decreased to 9%
in the 1990s. Reduction of the claims for inadequate ventilation and esophageal
intubation accounted for nearly the entire decrease in brain damage or death from
the 1980s to the 1990s. All other causes remained relatively stable [10].

When claims are grouped as to which monitors were used during anesthesia,
the significance of the monitors begins to be seen. Comparing the 1990s to the
1980s, inadequate ventilation decreased significantly when either a pulse oximeter or capnograph was used. The pulse oximeter did not affect the proportion of
claims of esophageal intubation, however, unless it was used with a capnograph.
The portion of claims for difficult intubation was unchanged by use of the pulse
oximeter and capnograph monitors. The overall reduction in respiratory-related
damaging events (25% reduced to 9%) seems to be related to inadequate ventilation and esophageal intubation, both of which were most affected by the use of
pulse oximeter and capnograph monitors.

Webb and colleagues [11] published data from the Australian incident monitoring study, in which the first 2000 incidents reported were analyzed with respect
to the role of monitors used during general anesthesia. In 52% of these cases a
monitor detected the incident first; oximetry (27%) and capnography (24%)
detected more than half the incidents. Electrocardiography (19%), blood pressure
(12%), low pressure circuit alarm (8%), and oxygen analyzer (4%) also were
mentioned as playing a role in detecting anesthesia incidents. A theoretical
analysis was performed to determine which monitor—if used on its own—would
reliably detect each incident. The incidents were categorized into 60 clinical
situations. Used on its own, the pulse oximeter theoretically would have detected
82% of applicable incidents. Capnograhy detected 55%, and in combination with
the pulse oximeter 88% of the incidents would have been detected. Addition of a
blood pressure monitor increased the detectable incidents to 93%, and using all
three monitors plus an oxygen analyzer increased the detectable incidents to
95%. This study begins to present data on the usefulness of monitors in detecting incidents that were thought to be somehow contrary to the safety of patients. The relationship among monitoring, patient safety, and overall outcome
had been born.

Cullen and colleagues [12] at the Massachusetts General Hospital used unanticipated intensive care unit admissions as an outcome measure to assess the
quality of anesthesia care in a large teaching hospital. After introduction of pulse

oximetry in all anesthetizing locations, the overall rate of unanticipated intensive care unit admissions—specifically the rate of unanticipated intensive care unit admissions to rule out myocardial infarction—decreased significantly. Although the use of pulse oximetry did show a decrease in unanticipated intensive care unit admissions and possibly an increase in patient safety, the author questioned the usefulness of unanticipated intensive care unit admissions as a generic screen for quality assurance.

Reporting on the analysis of 1097 anesthesia-related closed claims malpractice actions, Tinker and colleagues [13] concluded that 314 incidents, nearly all of which resulted in death or brain damage, could have been prevented by the use of pulse oximetry or a combination of pulse oximetry and capnography. With this study the anesthesia community saw an increase in the evidence of the relationship between monitors and patient safety.

Before and after the introduction of monitoring standards at the hospitals of the Harvard Department of Anesthesia, Eichhorn [14] analyzed the incidence of severe anesthesia-related injury. Out of 757,000 procedures in which anesthesia was used between 1976 and 1985, 10 resulted in severe intraoperative accidents. Between 1985 and 1988, after monitoring standards had been established, only 1 accident out of 244,000 cases was seen. Two important conclusions were drawn. Although the data suggest that routine monitoring could help decrease anesthesia-related morbidity, it would take a prohibitively large number of patients to show any statistical significance.

In March 1993, Moller and colleagues [15,16] led a group from Denmark in the publication of the only large scale, randomized clinical trial of pulse oximetry. They studied the influence of pulse oximetry monitoring in the operating room and Post-Anesthesia Care Unit (PACU) on frequency of unanticipated perioperative events, changes in patient care, and the rate of postoperative complications. The study involved 20,802 adult patients who received general or regional anesthesia and were scheduled for elective or emergent noncardiac or non-neurosurgical procedures. During anesthesia and in the PACU, there was a 19-fold increase in the diagnosis of hypoxemia in the oximetry group. Similarly, in the operating room and PACU, an increased detection of hypoventilation, endobronchial intubation, bronchospasm, and atelectasis in the oximetry group was linked with the increased detection of hypoxemia. Likewise, the data analysis showed a significant reduction in the incidence of myocardial ischemia.

As one would expect, the oximetry group was associated with the diagnosis and correction of perioperative respiratory incidents and a reduction in myocardial ischemia. The oximetry and control groups did not differ with respect to cardiovascular, respiratory, neurologic, or infectious complications, however. Despite the possibility of increased patient safety and the successes of pulse oximetry in general, it did not affect the overall patient outcome. Likewise, capnography has been shown to be useful in detecting earlier the type of incidents thought to be most harmful during anesthesia [10]. Evidence from large scale randomized studies that show the ability of any monitor to improve outcome is noticeably lacking.

Brain function monitoring

More recently, the use of cerebral function monitors to assess depth of anesthesia and possibly affect outcome has reached national attention. Introduction of this monitor to the operating room has been reported to improve the anesthesia providers' ability to administer anesthetic drugs, decrease emergent times, and improve patient outcome by earlier discharge from the PACU and the ambulatory facility [17,18]. Examination of the evidence is paramount to understanding if cerebral function monitors have any impact on patient outcomes and safety.

One reason that cerebral function monitors are used in the operating room is to prevent intraoperative awareness. Awareness under general anesthesia is a frightening and complex experience for patients that can result in serious emotional injury and posttraumatic stress disorder. The frequency of anesthesia awareness has been found in multiple studies to range between 0.1% and 0.2% of all patients undergoing general anesthesia [19]. With approximately 21 million patients annually in the United States undergoing surgery and anesthesia, the occurrence ranges from 20,000 to 40,000 cases of awareness each year. Of the several cerebral function monitors cuurently on the market in the United States, only the BIS monitor (Aspect Medical Systems, Newton, Massachusetts) has been shown in clinical studies to help clinicians reduce the incidence of awareness with recall.

Ekman and colleagues [20] examined a prospective cohort of 4945 consecutive surgical patients in whom muscle relaxants were used in the conduction of general anesthesia. Patients were monitored with a BIS monitor, and intraoperative values were kept between 40 and 60. Patients were subsequently interviewed on three occasions for the occurrence of explicit recall. The BIS-monitored group was compared with a historical group of 7826 similar patients in whom no cerebral function monitoring was used. Compared with this control group, the BIS-monitored group showed a 77% reduction in the incidence of explicit recall.

Myles and colleagues [21] and the B-Aware trial group in Australia studied 2463 patients in a prospective, randomized, double-blind multicenter trial. Adult patients at high risk for awareness were randomized to a BIS-guided (1225 patients) or routine practice (1238 patients) general anesthesia. Patients were assessed using a blinded observer at 2 to 6 hours, 24 to 36 hours, and 30 days after surgery. An independent committee, which was blinded to group identity, assessed each report of awareness. There were two reports of awareness in the BIS-guided group and 11 reports of awareness in the routine group. BIS-guided anesthesia reduced the risk of awareness by 82%.

Early data such as these last two studies have prompted national organizations to promote methods to reduce the incidence of awareness and increase patient safety in the population. On October 6, 2004, the Joint Commission on Accreditation of Health Care Organizations issued a sentinel event alert [22]. They noted that the US Food and Drug Administration had determined that "use of BIS monitoring to help guide anesthetic administration may be associated with the reduction of the incidence of awareness with recall in adults undergoing general anesthesia and sedation." The Joint Commission recommended that hospitals that perform procedures under general anesthesia develop and implement an anesthetic awareness policy that includes education of staff about awareness, identification of high-risk patients, effective use of anesthesia monitoring techniques, appropriate postoperative follow-up, and management strategies to help patients who experience intraoperative awareness.

In October 2005, the American Society of Anesthesiologists House of Delegates approved a "Practice Advisory for Intraoperative Awareness and Brain Function Monitoring" [23]. In it they recommended the assessment of risk for each patient and the use of a brain function monitor on a case-by-case basis to help in the prevention of intraoperative awareness. Although cerebral function monitors have not been granted the same status as monitors included in the standards for basic anesthesia monitoring, regulatory agencies, industry, and the public have brought the use of cerebral function monitors to the forefront in decreasing intraoperative awareness and increasing patient safety.

Aside from the topic of awareness, cerebral function monitors also have been shown to contribute to better postoperative outcomes. Significant benefits coming from multiple studies suggest that titrating anesthetic administration to the target organ—the brain—can produce less patient acuity in the PACU. Other studies have raised the possibility of long-term outcome benefits from cerebral function monitors.

Wong and colleagues [24] at the University of Toronto studied 68 patients over the age of 60. Patients were randomized to two groups: BIS titrated to a value between 50 and 60 and a standard practice group. The study was designed to investigate the effects of BIS monitoring on recovery profiles, level of postoperative cognitive dysfunction, and anesthetic drug requirements in elderly patients who were undergoing general anesthesia for orthopedic surgery. Although there was no difference in postoperative cognitive dysfunction between the two groups, the total isoflurane usage was 30% lower and recovery was significantly faster in the BIS group.

Nelskyla and colleagues [25] tested the hypothesis that monitoring with the BIS monitor decreases the incidence and severity of postoperative nausea and vomitting (PONV) and improves recovery and home readiness after outpatient gynecologic surgery. Patients were randomized to two groups: BIS titrated to a value between 50 and 60 and a control group with no BIS. Both groups received propofol induction followed by sevoflurane in 65% nitrous oxide and oxygen. The sevoflurane was titrated in the control group to keep hemodynamic variables within 25% of control values. Orientation and early recovery were achieved earlier in the BIS group, and patients performed better in the psychomotor recovery tests. The BIS group also had significantly less PONV (16% versus 40%) compared with the control group. No differences were found in times to achieve home readiness, however, probably because of the requirement by this institution that the patient void before discharge, which is a practice that is currently thought to be unnecessary in most modern ambulatory surgical suites.

In a large meta-analysis of randomized, controlled trials, Liu [26] examined the use of BIS monitoring versus standard practice in 1380 ambulatory patients from 11 different trials. BIS monitoring significantly reduced anesthetic use by 19%, reduced the incidence of PONV (32%, versus standard practice 38%), and reduced the time in recovery by an average of 4 minutes. No difference was seen in patient discharge times.

Although long-term outcome data are lacking in these studies, short-term benefits in areas such as PONV and early recovery times have been seen. Is it correct to say that patients are safer from the immediate postoperative effects of general anesthesia? In answering this question, one should review the data from a key preliminary observational study conducted at the Medical College of Georgia.

The study was designed to identify any impact of adding routine cerebral function monitoring to the operating rooms of the Medical College of Georgia. Data from two groups were collected prospectively. Group 1 consisted of 1515 patients who received general anesthesia in standard practice format. Group 2 consisted of 1191 patients who had standard practice plus BIS monitor titration of general anesthesia. This study involved a sequential trial in which group 1 patients underwent surgery first, then BIS monitors were put into each operating room and data collected for group 2 patients. The hypothesis was that in addition to early postoperative recovery, cerebral function monitoring would show benefits in the improvement of patient acuity in the PACU. In this large sequential clinical experience, the routine use of cerebral function monitoring was associated with faster postoperative recovery, increase in PACU bypass frequency, and decrease in PACU length of stay. Along with the significant decreases in recovery times, group 2 patients also experienced fewer postoperative side effects from surgery and anesthesia. Group 2 patients had significantly fewer cardiovascular, pain, and PONV issues [27].

Although data concerning administration of narcotics, beta-blockers, and inhalational anesthetics in this observational study were not collected, the authors hypothesized that by titrating the inhalational anesthetics to a BIS range of 45 to 60, other adjuvants were increasingly necessary to control for perturbations in patient intraoperative hemodynamics. Clinicians would use more narcotics and beta-blockers to blunt the surgical responses to painful stimuli (ie, increases in blood pressure, heart rate, and respiratory rate). It would stand to reason that patients in group 2 who received less inhalational anesthesia and more narcotics and beta-blockers would have fewer pain, cardiovascular, and PONV issues in the PACU. This study demonstrated that using cerebral function monitors would increase patient safety from common postoperative side effects in the early recovery phase.

Although little is known about the overall impact of monitors on patient safety, even less is known about the effect of anesthetic management on long-term outcomes. One controversial study brought to light the possibility that anesthetic management (cumulative deep hypnotic time) with the use of cerebral function monitors was an independent predictor of increased mortality within 1 year.

Monk and colleagues [28] at the University of Florida designed a prospective observational study of adult patients undergoing major noncardiac surgery with general anesthesia to determine if mortality in the first year after surgery was associated with demographic, preoperative clinical, surgical, or intraoperative variables. A total of 1064 patients aged 18 and older were enrolled in the study. One-year mortality rate was 5.5% in all patients and 10.3% in patients aged 65 or older. Most deaths were attributable to cancer (51.7%) and cardiovascular causes (17.2%). Analysis of the data identified three variables as significant independent projectors of mortality: patient comorbidity, cumulative deep hypnotic time, and intraoperative systolic hypotension. It is easy to understand why comorbidity was found as a significant predictor, because one would think that the sicker a patient is, the greater the mortality. Likewise, intraoperative hypotension may be related to myocardial dysfunction, sepsis, or hypovolemina, but a separate study is required for validation. It may be difficult to understand how cumulative deep hypnotic time could influence 1 -year mortality, however. One explanation for this finding could be related to the effects that volatile anesthetic agents have on the immune system and how they might influence progression of pre-existing chronic diseases [29–33]. Cerebral function monitors have been shown in multiple studies to reduce the amount of anesthesia given, and in light of this study they may be implicated in greater patient safety and decreased mortality. Clearly this subject is controversial but highly intriguing, and it demands further study.

Summary

There is much more to study and learn about prevention of anesthesia complications and how technology may improve the safety and outcome of anesthesia. Large trials have never shown that a specific hemodynamic monitoring technique improves outcome. In controlled situations, oximetry and capnography have demonstrated efficacy in early detection of events that could be harmful during anesthesia. The BIS monitor has been shown to affect early recovery outcomes and possibly be of value in decreasing long-term mortality. Through all the controversy one thing remains constant: the response to information coming from monitors depends solely on the person administering the anesthesia. Aids to practitioner vigilance probably can never be proved to possess independent benefit, but their role in improving practitioner performance cannot be argued.

References

[1] Beecher HK, Todd DP. A study of the deaths associated with anesthesia and surgery. Ann Surg 1954;140:2–34.
[2] Dripps RD, Lamont A, Eckenhoff JE. The role of anesthesia in surgical mortality. JAMA 1961;178:261–6.
[3] Phillips OC, Frazier TM, Graff TD, et al. The Baltimore anesthesia study committee. JAMA 1960;174:2015–9.

[4] Lunn JN, Mushin WW. Mortality associated with anesthesia. London: Nuffield Provincial Hospitals Trust; 1982.

[5] Anesthesia Patient Safety Foundation Newsletter. Groups publish conventions. Available at: www.apsf.org. Accessed November 2005.

[6] Eichhorn JH, Cooper JR, Cullen DJ, et al. Standards for patient monitoring during anesthesia at Harvard Medical School. JAMA 1986;256:1017–20.

[7] American Society of Anesthesiology. Monitoring standards of care: history of the ASA. Available at: www.ASAhq.org. Accessed November 2005.

[8] Pierce BC. The establishment of the APSF and the ASA closed claims study: the 34th Rovenstine lecture. Available at: www.APSF.org. Accessed November 2005.

[9] Cheney FW. ASA closed claims project: where have we been and where are we going? American Society of Anesthesiologists Newsletter 1993;57:8–22.

[10] Cheney FW. Changing trends in anesthesia: related death and permanent brain damage. American Society of Anesthesiologists Newsletter 2002;66(6):6–8.

[11] Webb RK, van der Walt JH, Runciman WB, et al. The Australian incident monitoring study: which monitor? An analysis of 200 incident reports. Anaesth Intensive Care 1993; 21(5):529–42.

[12] Cullen DJ, Nemeskal AR, Cooper JB, et al. Effect of pulse oximetry, age, and ASA physical status on the frequency of patients admitted unexpectedly to the postoperative intensive care unit and the severity of their anesthesia-related complications. Anesth Analg 1992;74:181–8.

[13] Tinker JH, Dull DL, Cuplan RA, et al. Role of monitoring devices in prevention of anesthesia mishaps: a closed claims study. Anesthesiology 1989;71:541–6.

[14] Eichhorn JH. Prevention of intraoperative anesthesia accidents and related severe injury through safety monitoring. Anesthesiology 1989;7:572–7.

[15] Moller JT, Johannessen NW, Espersen K, et al. Randomized evaluation of pulse oximetry in 20,802 patients: II. perioperative events and postoperative complications. Anesthesiology 1993; 78:445–53.

[16] Moller JT, Pederson T, et al. Randomized evaluation of 20,802 patients: 1 design demography, pulse oximetry failure rate and overall complication rate. Anesthesiology 1993;78:436–44.

[17] Wong J, Song D, Blanshard H, et al. Titration of isoflurane using BIS index improves early recovery of elderly patients undergoing orthopedic surgeries. Can J Anesth 2002;49(1):13–8.

[18] Gan TJ, Glass PS, Windsor A, et al, and the BIS Utility Study Group. Bispectral index monitoring allows faster emergence and improved recovery from propofol, alfentanil, and nitrous oxide anesthesia. Anesthesiology 1997;87(4):808–15.

[19] Sebel PS, Bowdle TA, Ghoneim MM, et al. The incidence of awareness during anesthesia: a multicenter United States study. Anesth Analg 2004;99:833–9.

[20] Ekman A, Lindholm ML, Lennmarken C, et al. Reduction in the incidence of awareness using BIS monitoring. Acta Anesthesiol Scand 2004;48(1):20–6.

[21] Myles PS, Leslie K, McNeil J, et al. Bispectral index monitoring to prevent awareness during anaesthesia: the B-aware randomized controlled trail. Lancet 2004;363:1757–63.

[22] JCAHO. Sentinel event alert issue. Available at: www.jcaho.org. Accessed November 2005.

[23] American Society of Anesthesiologists. Report by the American Society of Anesthesiologists Task Force on Intraoperative Awareness. Available at: www.ASAhq.org. Accessed November 2005.

[24] Wong J, Song D, Blanshard H, et al. Titration of isoflurane using BIS index improves early recovery of elderly patients undergoing orthopedic surgery. Can J Anesth 2002;49:13–8.

[25] Nelskyla KA, Yli-Hankala AM, Puro HP, et al. Sevoflurane titration using bispectral index decreases postoperative vomiting in phase II recovery after ambulatory surgery. Anesth Analg 2001;93:1165–9.

[26] Liu SS. Effects of bispectral index monitoring on ambulatory anesthesia: a meta-analysis of randomized controlled trials and a cost analysis. Anesthesiology 2004;101:311–5.

[27] Mayfield JB, Meiler SE, Head CA. Routine cerebral function monitoring improves postoperative acuity and recovery from general anesthesia [abstract]. Anesthesiology 2004;101:A291.

[28] Monk TG, Saini V, Weldon CB, et al. Anesthetic management and one-year mortality after noncardiac surgery. Anesth Analg 2004;100(1):4–10.

[29] Meiler SE, Monk TG, Mayfield JB, et al. Can we alter long-term outcome? The role of anesthetic management and the inflammatory response. APSF Newsletter 2003;18(3):33,35,37.

[30] Meiler SE, Monk TG, Mayfield JB, et al. Can we alter long-term outcome? The role of inflammation and immunity in the perioperative period (Part II). APSF Newsletter 2004;19(1): 1,3,4,7.

[31] Lennmarken C, Lindholm M, Greenwald S, et al. Confirmation that low intraoperative BIS levels predict increased risk of postoperative mortality. Anesthesiology 2003;99:A303.

[32] Greenwald S, Sandin R, Lindholm M, et al. Prolonged low intraoperative BIS levels predict increased risk of postoperative mortality: two-year follow up report. Anesthesiology 2004; 101:A384.

[33] Greenwald S, Sandin R, Lindholm M, et al. Duration at low intraoperative BIS levels was shorter among one-year postoperative survivors than non-survivors: a case-controlled analysis. Anesthesiology 2004;101:A383.

ELSEVIER
SAUNDERS

Anesthesiology Clin N Am
24 (2006) 419–425

ANESTHESIOLOGY
CLINICS OF
NORTH AMERICA

Index

Note: Page numbers of article titles are in **boldface** type.

0889-8537/06/$ – see front matter © 2006 Elsevier Inc. All rights reserved.
doi:10.1016/S0889-8537(06)00032-0 *anesthesiology.theclinics.com*

Changing Your Address?

Make sure your subscription changes too! When you notify us of your new address, you can help make our job easier by including an exact copy of your Clinics label number with your old address (see illustration below.) This number identifies you to our computer system and will speed the processing of your address change. Please be sure this label number accompanies your old address and your corrected address—you can send an old Clinics label with your number on it or just copy it exactly and send it to the address listed below.

We appreciate your help in our attempt to give you continuous coverage. Thank you.

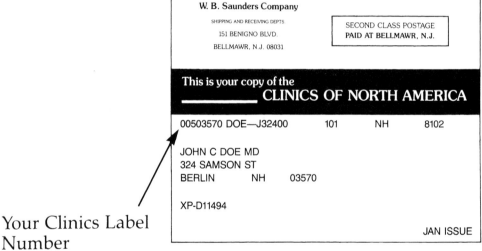

W. B. Saunders Company

SHIPPING AND RECEIVING DEPTS.
151 BENIGNO BLVD.
BELLMAWR, N.J. 08031

SECOND CLASS POSTAGE
PAID AT BELLMAWR, N.J.

This is your copy of the
_____ CLINICS OF NORTH AMERICA

00503570 DOE—J32400   101   NH   8102

JOHN C DOE MD
324 SAMSON ST
BERLIN   NH   03570

XP-D11494

JAN ISSUE

Your Clinics Label Number
Copy it exactly or send your label along with your address to:
W.B. Saunders Company, Customer Service
Orlando, FL 32887-4800
Call Toll Free 1-800-654-2452

Please allow four to six weeks for delivery of new subscriptions and for processing address changes.